Acupuncture for Emergencies

Martin Wang
MD., Ph.D, R. Acupuncturist

© 2017 Martin Wang
All rights reserved.

ISBN: 1975686446
ISBN 13: 9781975686444
Library Control of Congress Number: 2018900381
CreateSpace Independent Publishing Platform, North Charleston, SC

Contents

Foreword 8
Note to Readers 10
Chapter 1 11
Introduction to the Therapies Commonly Used 11
in Emergency Conditions 11
   Acupuncture 11
   Location of Acupun cture Point 11
   Choice of Needle 13
   Deepness of Needle 14
   Acupuncture Sensation 15
   Time the Needle Is Kept in the Skin 15
   Sterilization 15
   Bleeding Therapy 15
   Moxibustion 16
   Tuina Massage 17
   Chinese Herbal Therapy 17
   Folk Therapy 18
Chapter 2 19
Acute Clinic Conditions 19
   Shock 19
   Coma 20
   Bleeding 21
      Bleeding Due to Trauma (beating, car accident, and so on) 21
      Internal Bleeding 22
      Bleeding from nose or gums 22
      Bleeding from the lung 22
      Bleeding from the stomach 23
      Bleeding from the intestine 23
      Bleeding from the urinary system 24
   Stroke 25
   High Fever 25
   Trauma 27
      Cerebral Concussion 27
      Trauma to Chest 27
      Trauma to Abdomen 28

- Trauma to Body Muscles 28
- Heart Disease 29
  - Myocardial Infarction and Angina Pectoris4 29
  - Heart Failure—When the Heart Is About to Stop Beating 30
- Panic Attack 30
- Epilepsy 30
- Hysteria 31
- Gynecology and Obstetrics 32
  - Bleeding from the Uterus 32
  - Dysmenorrhea 32
  - Fetus Malposition 33
  - Expedite Fetus Delivery 34
  - Retained Placenta 34
  - Nocturnal Fretfulness in Infants 34
- Burns (Fire, Boiling Water, and Similar) 35
- Frostbite 36
- Drowning 38
- Heatstroke 42
- Carbon Monoxide Toxicity 43
- Acute and Heavy Dizziness 44
- Acute Pain on the Body's Surface 44
  - Migraine 44
  - Trigeminal Neuralgia 45
  - Bell's Palsy 45
  - Headache Due to High Blood Pressure 46
  - Neck Stiffness 46
  - Acute Shoulder Pain 47
  - Acute Pain on the Elbow 48
  - Acute Wrist Pain 49
  - Acute Back Pain 49
  - Acute Sciatic Pain 51
  - Acute Tailbone Pain 52
  - Acute Knee Pain 53
  - Calf Spasm 54
  - Acute Bruise on the Ankle 54
  - Acute Pain on the Heel 55
  - Foot Pain 56

- Gout 56
- Herpes Zoster 58
- Acute Pain in the Mouth, Throat, or Abdomen 59
  - Toothache 59
  - Mouth Ulcer 60
  - Acute Pain in the Throat 61
  - Acute Mumps 62
  - Acute Gastritis 62
  - Gastric Ulcer 64
  - Acute Appendicitis 65
  - Acute Gallstones 65
  - Roundworm in Gallbladder 65
  - Acute Kidney Stone 66
  - Acute Intestinal Obstruction or Enteroparalysis 66
  - Incarcerated Hernia 66
  - Hemorrhoids 67
- Heavy Cough 68
- Hiccups 70
- Aphonia 71
- Nausea and Vomiting 72
  - Due to Pregnancy 72
  - Due to Car Sickness (or Plane Sickness or Boat Sickness) 72
  - Due to Gastric Disorders 72
- Acute Constipation 74
- Acute Diarrhea 74
- Acute Urinary Retention 76
- Fishbone Stuck in Throat 77
- Heavy Asthma 78
- Common Cold or Flu 79
- Bites by Animals or Insects 81
  - Bites by Bees or Other Insects 81
  - Bites by Snakes 82
  - Bites by Dogs or Other Animals 83
- Drunkenness 83
- Foreign Matter in the Ear 84

Chapter 3 85
List of Acupuncture Points 85

Chapter 4 Acupuncture Points Figures..115
Alphabetic index..128
Our Publications..131
References 132

Foreword

This book is intended to be a handbook for acupuncture treatment used in emergency conditions. I've tried to make the contents as simple as possible, allowing users to find the proper treatment for each condition without explaining the reasons for using these therapies and these acupuncture points. If a reader is interested in knowing more details about acupuncture, I recommend consulting more professional books.

Acupuncture is one of the most powerful therapies in Chinese medicine. In this handbook, I mostly introduce acupuncture. Chinese herbal therapy is another powerful therapy for emergency. It needs the practitioner to have a higher level of knowledge about herbal therapy and a rich clinical experience in using it. For this reason, herbal therapy is only mentioned briefly. I also introduce some Tuina techniques, not the point-injection technique, auricular acupuncture, or acupuncture point-imbedding therapy. Acupuncture is best done by hand, although it can also be performed by a machine (electrical acupuncture).

The information in this handbook should be useful for doctors in hospital emergency departments or clinics, physiotherapists, chiropractors, lifeguards, firefighters, outdoor travelers, military personnel, or any other person who might encounter an emergency health crisis. It is useful even for acupuncturists who had their acupuncture education in the West, because many of the techniques introduced in this handbook are beyond the contents of acupuncture textbooks. For more information about acupuncture and various other kinds of Chinese medicine, please refer to our other book, *More Than Acupuncture* (Friesenpress, 2018).

I recommend that these acupuncture techniques for emergent conditions be included in training courses for medical professionals who meet people in emergency conditions, including professional doctors, physiotherapists, or chiropractic practitioners. Conventional lifesaving techniques are not always perfect or sufficient. For example, in Chinese medicine, it is still possible to save the life of a drowned person even if the person "died" several hours earlier. Surely this is hardly explained by conventional medical knowledge about human life.

I also recommend having at least one acupuncturist in each emergency department. If the diagnosis for an emergency condition has been made, or if the diagnosis is hard to make, try acupuncture to stop the symptoms or to stop further development of the disease. The emergency room doctors should attempt to stop the disease as soon as possible, not let the patient wait for the next day to see another doctor or family physician. Just giving patients painkillers and letting them visit their family doctors the next day will not only prolong their suffering from the pain (many times the painkiller does not work properly), but it also will increase healthcare costs nationally.

The "emergency condition" in this book refers to any condition that makes people rush to the emergency department for medical help. Such conditions can be a stroke, heavy bleeding, trauma, a common cold with a fever, or an acute onset of chronic asthma.

In order to keep the content as brief and straightforward as possible, all the references are provided in reference list, instead of within the text.

Martin Wang, MD (China), PhD (Sweden)
Millwoods Acupuncture Center
Edmonton, Canada
August 20, 2017

Note to Readers

The information in this book has actually collected, cited and compiled from various sources. The contribution of the author is the English translation only. The book is intended to provide helpful and informative materials on the topics addressed in the publication. It is being sold with the understanding that the author is not engaged in rendering medical, health, or any other kind of personal or professional services in the book. The reader should consult his or her doctor or other competent health professional before adopting any of the suggestions in this book or drawing inferences from it. The author specifically disclaims all responsibility for any liability, loss, or risk, personal or otherwise, that is incurred as a consequence, directly or indirectly, of the use and application of any of the contents of this book.

Most of the information is collected from online and many times it is hard to find the name of the original authors or to contact the authors. If readers find that your information is cited but the source is not listed, or if you do not want the information cited, please contact me via e-mail (wenqiw57@hotmail.com). I will correct the mistake as soon as possible.

Chapter 1
Introduction to the Therapies Commonly Used in Emergency Conditions

Acupuncture

Acupuncture means to insert a special needle into the body to stimulate the body for treatment. An acupuncture point is a spot on the skin that Chinese medicine believes to have more life energy. To stimulate a different spot will have a different healing effect. The location of the spot is not the same from person to person and not the same for a given person between a healthy condition and a disease condition. In this handbook, I ask the reader to use the location of the spot as a reference; it is needed to find the tender place around the location of the acupuncture point.

Location of Acupun cture Point

To find the correct location of an acupuncture point, use the "same-body scale." It uses a mark from the given person's body. The commonly used way is with the finger, hands, and the local part of the body:

1. As shown in figure 1, the lines between the second stem of the index finger equal one cun (cun is a unit in Chinese scale).
2. The distance across the four fingers of a hand is measured from the level of the first line on the back of the index finger.
3. The scale in each part of the body. For example, the distance from the wrist line to the elbow line (the palm side) is twelve cun, the distance between the external malleolus and the out sunken of the knee is sixteen cun, the distance from the navel to the symphysis ossium pubis is five cun, the distance from under the cartilago ensiformis to the navel is eight cun, the distance between the two nipples is eight cun, and so on.

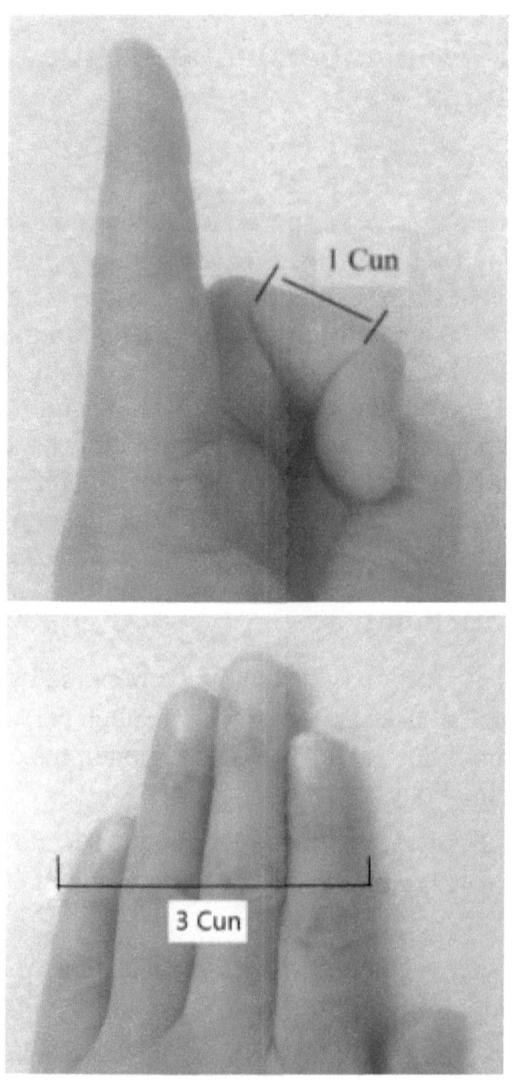

Figure 1. Same-body scale for acupuncture (on finger)

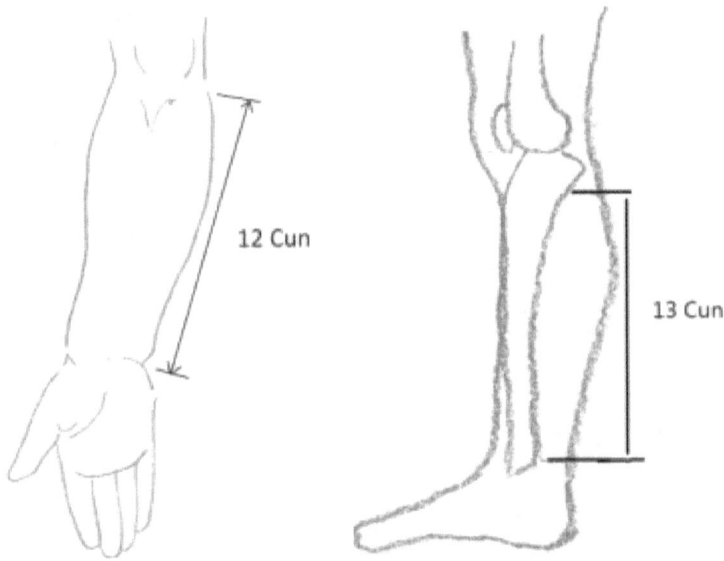

Figure 2. Same-body scale for acupuncture (on arm and leg)

Choice of Needle

The needle used in an emergency condition usually needs to be hard and relatively thick. I commonly use 0.30 millimeter (mm) by 50 mm or 0.35 mm by 75 mm. However, needles of other sizes can be used. If there is no proper needle, you can use any sharp material, such as a suture needle, a paper clip, or even a longer thorn from a tree. In an emergency condition, the life is in danger, and any means can be used to save the life.

Needles can be purchased from Chinese herbal stores. They can be found by a Google search using key words of "acupuncture," "supply," and "needles."

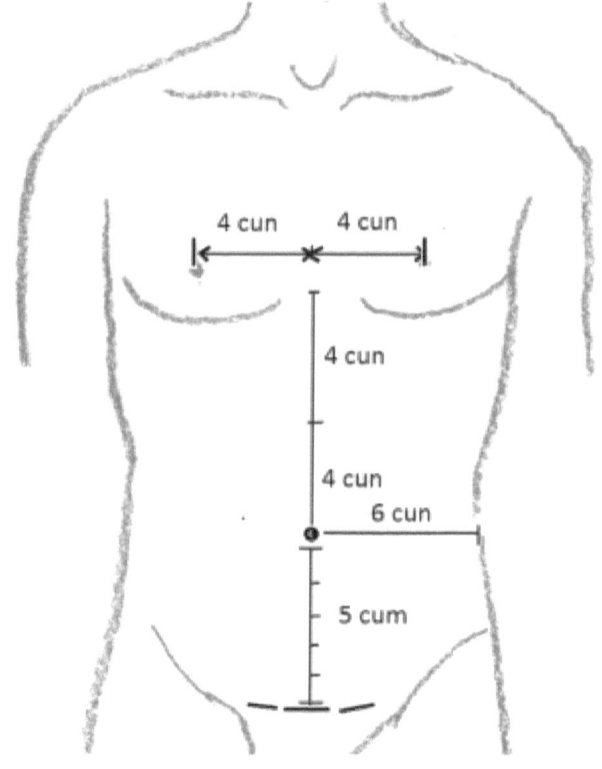

Figure 3. Same-body scale for acupuncture (on chest and abdomen)

Deepness of Needle

The deepness of a needle in the body depends on the part of the body. Basically, for a needle in the scalp, it is horizontal with an angle of about fifteen degrees to the scalp skin. It is mostly in a declining angle of about fifteen to twenty-five degrees to the skin, when used in the chest and back (with the needle tips away from the spine). In most of the other parts of the body, it is vertical. But in the abdomen, insert the needle down until you can feel a slight resistance. It means that the needle touches the peritoneum. Do not penetrate deeper into the abdomen.

For an obese person, the needle is inserted deeper. For a slim person, needle insertion is shallow.

Acupuncture Sensation

Usually it is best to allow the person have a special feeling after insertion of the needle. It is called acupuncture sensation or *Deqi*. It is a kind of tingling, numbness, slight bloating, or painful feeling under the needle. If the patient is in shock or a coma, it is impossible to know if the patient has such a feeling or not. The operator needs to feel a light tightness under the skin and some pulling feeling to attract the needle. This is another way to get the acupuncture sensation. In an emergency condition, the needle is twisted or pulled and inserted with relatively stronger force (compared to the treatment of a chronic condition). Such a *Deqi* sensation is not difficult to obtain.

Time the Needle Is Kept in the Skin

The needle is usually kept in the skin for 20 to 30 minutes (min). For the treatment of shock or coma, it may be kept for a longer time until the condition is clearly improved. For acute pain, it is quickly inserted and quickly taken away after the pain has subsided (it may need several min only).

Sterilization

In routine clinic work, disinfect the skin with 75 percent alcohol before the insertion of the needle. However, in an emergency condition, and especially if the emergency occurs outdoors, it is impossible to have this procedure. Try to clean the skin of the person and the hands of the operator with clear or pure water or similar before acupuncture.

Bleeding Therapy

Bleeding therapy means to remove some amount of blood from the body. In some cases, this is a very efficient therap and is used before acupuncture. There is large-volume bleeding therapy, which is used in the treatment of varicose veins, and small-volume bleeding therapy, in which only several drops of blood are released out of the body. In emergency treatment, the small-volume bleeding therapy is usually used.

Skin with clear veins can be stabbed with a lancet or a Chinese triangle-edged needle.

After release of some drops of blood, the bleeding spot is covered with a cup (used in a cupping therapy) until no blood comes out of the skin or until the color of the blood turns fresh red.

Moxibustion

Moxibustion means to stimulate the acupuncture point or an affected skin area with heat from burning herbs. The herbs used for such aim are called moxi. It can be a shape of a roll (about twenty centimeters long), a cone, or a cylinder. There are direct (the moxi touches the skin) or indirect (the moxi does not touch the skin) ways of moxibustion. For the indirect way, burn a moxi roll at one end, hold it over the treated skin with several centimeters of distance, and move it in a line or circle to let the skin feel warm but not burning. It is used for about 30 min or until the skin turns pink in color (figure 4). Another way is to put a thin layer of fresh ginger on the treated skin (or acupuncture point) and then to put a cone-shaped moxi on the ginger and burn it until the skin feels very hot (figure 5). Direct moxibustion means to put a moxi cone directly on the skin, to burn it, and to remove it when the patient feels very hot from the burning cone. In an emergency condition, the most often used is the indirect way.

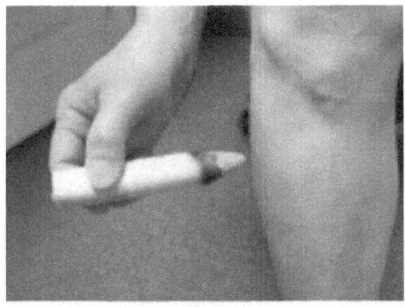

Figure 4. Indirect moxibustion on leg

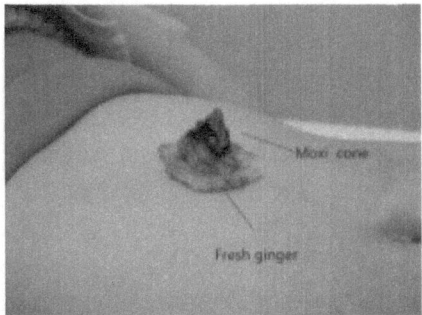

Figure 5. Indirect moxibustion (with fresh ginger on the skin)

Tuina Massage

Tuina is a kind of Chinese medicine massage technique. It is mostly used in emergency conditions for the treatment of pain syndrome.

Chinese Herbal Therapy

Chinese herbal therapy is one of the most powerful therapies in Chinese medicine. I have introduced some herbal formulas in this handbook. I recommend that the clinic or emergency room keep some of the herbal formulas on hand in case they are needed. The herbal formulas are now in ready-to-use granule form. To use, just take two to three teaspoons (about

2 to 4 grams (g)), dissolve it in water, and give it to the patient to drink. It can be repeated once every two to three hours until the body condition becomes stable.

If the patient is in shock or in a coma and cannot drink, deliver it directly to the stomach with a stomach tube. This is a very important therapy, especially (a) to reduce extremely high fever (this condition is frequently seen in hospitals) and (b) to increase blood pressure in shock and drowning patients. These are just a few examples.

Folk Therapy

Folk therapies are the ways ordinary people in China used to treat diseases or discomfort. The recipes are tested by the people themselves, not by Chinese medicine doctors, though the doctors might also use them in clinics. In many cases, these recipes work well if they are used in a proper way. I will cite some of the recipes here in case the professional services from either Western medicine or Chinese medicine are not available. There are many recipes, but the ones cited in this book are chosen for the consideration of the availability of the materials or the ingredients in the Western countries. However, we still recommend readers consult with Chinese medicine doctors before using them.

Chapter 2
Acute Clinic Conditions

Shock

1. Use acupuncture on the DU26 point (needle tip is declining toward the top of the head) (figure 6).

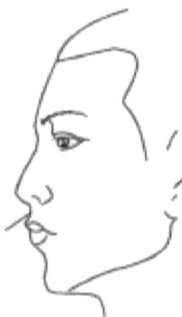

Figure 6. The needle on the DU26 point should be toward the top of the head.

2. Use acupuncture on the DU25 (needle is toward the top of the head), PC6, and KID1 points, plus two or three of the following points: DU26, ST36, DU20, LI4, and Shixuan. Retain the needles for one to twelve hours or until the blood pressure is stable.
3. Use acupuncture on the DU23 (penetrating to the DU20 point) and ST36 points.
4. Finger press the PC6, LU11, LI4, ST36, and DU26 points.
5. Use moxibustion on the REN4, REN17, DU20, and REN6 points for 15 to 30 min.

Note:
1. Perform acupuncture first, with or without moxibustion therapy.

2. Twist the needles every 15 to 20 min. Electric acupuncture can be used.
3. When the DU26 point is pressed with the finger, do not press for too long a time; press it as a wave to avoid damage to the skin.
4. Acupuncture and moxibustion work for any type of shock (cardiac shock, infectious shock, hypovolemic shock, toxic shock, traumatic shock, or allergic shock).
5. Acupuncture therapy should be combined with conventional therapies.
6. It has been found that the acupuncture used in the treatment of various types of shock has the following benefits:
    - Blood pressure can gradually increase within 4 to 30 min (faster than conventional therapies).
    - The lower the blood pressure is before acupuncture, the faster the blood pressure increases.
    - Acupuncture still works even if pressure agents alone fail.
    - Acupuncture can increase blood pressure, enhance heartbeat, improve breathing, increase urine volume, increase blood sugar level, and more.

All suggest that acupuncture can work to stabilize the inner life environment. The overall efficiency of acupuncture in the treatment of shock averages more than 85 percent.

Coma

1. Use acupuncture on the DU26, PC9, KID1, and ST36 points, plus one or two of the following points: LI4, LU11, SI3, PC8, and PC6.
2. Use bleeding therapy on the DU20 point.

3. Use bleeding therapy on the LU11, hand Shixuan, feet Shixuan,[1] and DU20 points (figure 7).
4. Use acupuncture on the DU20 and KID1 points.
5. Use acupuncture on the Brain-wake point.
6. Use acupuncture on the Paralysis point.

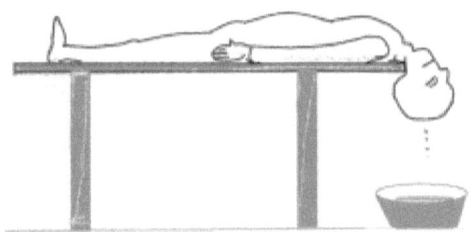

Figure 7. Body posture when bleeding therapy is used on the DU20 point. The head falls down the edge of the bed.

Bleeding

Bleeding Due to Trauma (beating, car accident, and so on)

1. For open wounds on the skin, use acupuncture on the two ends of the wound to stop bleeding.
2. Use bleeding therapy on the KID2, ST42, and Three-hair points.
3. Use acupuncture on the GB21 and ST36 points.
4. Use acupuncture on a point depending on meridians.
5. Use these herbal teas: Guizhi Tang plus Taoren (for trauma in muscle), Sini San (for trauma on abdomen[2] or chest), or Sanhuang Xiexin Tang.

---

1. It is on the tips of the toes on both feet.
2. If there is bleeding in the abdomen, there is pressing pain on the lower abdomen, about three cun to the left side of the REN4 point.

6. Use folk therapy for bleeding due to knife cuts or other kinds of cuts. Materials: 60 g of litchi core and 60 g of dried longan culp (Guiyuan rou). Grind the two into powder, and apply to the bleeding spot.

Internal Bleeding
Bleeding from nose or gums
1. Use acupuncture on the LU3 point (on healthy side).
2. Use acupuncture on the Xiabai point (on healthy side).
3. Use acupuncture on the LU11 point (on sick side).
4. Use acupuncture on the ST44 point.
5. Use folk therapy.
    - For nosebleeds. Put a cotton ball in vinegar. Take it out, and apply into the nose.
    - For nosebleeds. Material: one cup Chinese chive juice. Drink it. In the summer, drink it after cooling it, and in the winter, drink it after warming it a little bit.
    - For nosebleeds. Material: 50 g Loquat leaves. Dry the leaves, and drink the powder with regular green tea from time to time. Repeat for several days.
    - For nosebleeds during menstrual periods. Materials: 100 mililiter (ml) fresh sugarcane juice, 100 ml fresh lotus juice, and 100 ml fresh *Rehmannia glutinosa libosch* (Shen Di) juice. Mix all well. Drink it when bleeding.
    - For gum bleeding. Material: tomato. Eat it as regular fruit, and continue for two weeks.

Bleeding from the lung
1. Use acupuncture on the LU6 and LIV13 points.
2. Use acupuncture on the Lung-ease point.

3. Use acupuncture on the LU7, LU5, UB13, LU10, LU9, LU6, and PC6 points.
4. Do flower-needle taping of the arteria cervicalis (up and down for 15 to 20 min).
5. Use folk therapy.

    - For cough with blood. Materials: 30 g banana skin, 30 g *Chrysanthemum indicum* (ye ju hua), and 20 g rock sugar. Add to water, and cook as a soup. Drink as a green tea every day.
    - For cough with blood. Materials: 30 g sugarcane skin, 30 g Yiming of the Senate (Sha shen), and 3 g mountain prickly ash (Wuweizi). Add all to water, and cook as a soup for 60 min. Drink it two to three times a day for several days.

Bleeding from the stomach

1. Use acupuncture on the UB17, UB21, PC6, and ST36 points.
2. Use folk therapy.

    - Chop garlic into mud (paste). Apply it on the bottom of the foot, fold with gauze, and keep for several hours.
    - Press cabbage to collect juice. Add a little white sugar in it. Drink the mixture every day, 30 ml each time. You can also drink it before each meal every day, 100 to 200 ml each time.
    - Use watermelon cane (100 g) and lotus flower (30 g). Add both to water, and cook as a soup. Drink the extract twice a day.

Bleeding from the intestine

1. Use acupuncture on the UB57, KID7, DU1, and Erbai points.
2. Use moxibustion on the DU20 point

3. Use folk therapy.
   - Dry several carrot leaves naturally in air. Grind them into powder. Drink the powder, 6 g each time, twice a day.
   - Burn eggplant (with its stems) into ash. Grind into powder. Drink 9 g of the powder; swallow with cooking wine (20 ml). Repeat for one week.
   - Materials: 30 g luffa (bake to black in color) and 30 g sophorae (Huai hua). Mix the materials, and grind them into powder. Drink the powder twice a day, 6 g each time.
   - Material: 90 g luffa cane. Bake 90 g of luffa cane until black in color. Grind into powder. Drink it twice a day with the addition of a little cooking wine.
   - Materials: one cup watermelon juice and 20 g brown sugar. Mix. Drink the mixture three times a day.

Bleeding from the urinary system

1. Use acupuncture on the UB23, UB28, SP9, SP10, and SP6 points.
2. Use herbal therapy of 60 g Baimaogen and 60 g Xianhecao. Cook in 1000 ml of water until the liquid left in the pot is about 600 ml. Drink 100 ml of the liquid extract every two hours.
3. Use folk therapy.
   - Use fresh celery to prepare juice. Drink the juice three times a day, 40 ml each time.
   - Use 15 g grape root and 15 g white sugar. Add the grape root to water, and boil for one hour. Collect the extract, and mix with the sugar. Drink the extract mixture every day. Repeat for several days.
   - Materials: 100 ml sugarcane juice and 15 g peach kernel. Add the peach kernel to water, and cook as a

soup for 60 min. Mix with the cane juice. Drink it once to twice a day for several days.

Note: For all kinds of bleeding, use acupuncture on the SP10 point.

Stroke

1. Use bleeding therapy on the veins on the back of the ears.
2. Use bleeding therapy on the DU20 and LU11 points.
3. Use bleeding therapy on the Shixuan points.
4. Use acupuncture on the DU26 point (especially for the treatment of anepia).
5. Use acupuncture on the REN23 point (patient lies face up) and DU15 point (patient lies face down).
6. Use acupuncture on the DU20 and KID1 points.
7. Use acupuncture on the GB8 and ST41 points.
8. Use acupuncture on the GB20 point (especially for cerebral ischemia).
9. Use acupuncture on the SJ18 point.
10. Use acupuncture on the Shoulder-back point (two cun away from the tailbone).

Note: In addition to the conventional treatment for stroke, acupuncture should be started as soon as possible to speed up the return to consciousness, to reduce the chance of inhalation of phlegm into the lung, to reduce brain damage, and to reduce later paralysis.

High Fever

For adult:

1. Use bleeding therapy on the veins on the back of the ears.

2. Use bleeding and cupping therapy on the DU14 point, and then use cupping on it.
3. Use bleeding therapy on the LU11 and LI1 points (especially f or acute tonsillitis).
4. Use acupuncture on the SJ5 point (deep to the PC6 point).
5. Use acupuncture on the LI11 point.

For children:
1. Use bleeding therapy on the LU11 and LI1 points.
2. Use Tian-he-shui Tuina technique.

    There are many Tuina massage therapies in Chinese medicine to solve diseases in children. The Tian-he-shui massage is one of them and is used for a child with a fever.

    (1) Press and push several times the skin on the palm side of the front arm (for example, the PC6 point). This means to "open" the Tian-He-Shui.[3]

    (2) Press and push the skin slightly from the far end of the front arm to the tip of the middle finger (palm side with the rest of the fingers bent) several times. Then bend the child's middle finger to touch the palm. Press the child's middle finger to his palm several times (the operator's finger does not touch the palm of the child). After the child starts to sweat, the fever starts to reduce. It usually needs about 5 to 10 min.

    If the body temperature is very high, the pushing manner starts from the elbow to the fingertip.

---

3. *Tian* here means "sky," *He* means "river," and *Shui* means "water." So it means to bring water from the sky to reduce the fever.

(3) If the fever is still there, and if the child's lips and face are blue in color (cold condition), push the index finger, the middle finger, and the third finger—all from the fingertip—to the PC6 point. If the child's lips and face are red in color (fire condition), push from the PC6 point to the fingertips.

(4) Press the PC6 point several times again to end the operation. This is a required step.

The fingertips are to press the skin very slightly. For a boy, use his left arm and hand. For a girl, use her right arm and hand.

Note: In addition to acupuncture, Chinese herbal therapy is another powerful choice to reduce fever.

Trauma

Cerebral Concussion

When a person falls from a high space or is beaten by something, causing cerebral concussion and loss of consciousness, use the following treatments:
1. Use bleeding therapy on the KID2 point.
2. Use bleeding therapy on the veins on the back of the ears.
3. Use acupuncture on the DU26, DU20, and KID1 points.
4. Use acupuncture on the UB11, UB10, and UB66 points.
5. Use acupuncture on the GB21 and ST36 points.

Trauma to Chest
1. Use acupuncture on the GB21 and ST36 points.
2. Use acupuncture on the Chest-pain point.

Trauma to Abdomen

1. Use acupuncture on the GB21 and ST36 points.
2. Use acupuncture on the Chest-pain point.

Trauma to Body Muscles

1. For the treatment of pain due to trauma on the head, arms, legs, and so on, refer to the corresponding chapters for the treatment of pain.
2. For acute bruises, if a cold compress is used, it should not be used more than 20 min. It is recommended to use moxibustion (indirect moxibustion, with the moxi not touching the skin) on the affected body area for as long as three to four hours. This is not for open wounds.
3. If the body falls to the ground due to a fall or a beating, have the person lie on the ground without movement for 10 to 15 min, and then gradually move the body. Sudden and quick getting up causes more damage.
4. If bone fractures are suspected, use the conventional ways (Western or Chinese) to fix the fractures before acupuncture.

   Note:
   1. If the trauma is on a muscle, give the herbal tea Guizhi Tang (or Xiao Chaihu Tang) plus the herbs Taoren and Honghua. If trauma is in the stomach, give an herbal tea of Sini San plus Taoren and Honghui. If trauma is in the bladder, and the person cannot pass urine, give Taohe Chengqi Tang.
   2. Use folk therapy for all kinds of trauma.
      - Wash spinach and press it to collect juice. Drink the juice two to three times a day, 150 ml each time.
      - Dry orange core, and grind it into powder. Eat 10 g each time with liquor to help swallow.

3. How to tell if there is blood stagnation or dead blood in the body:
   - There is pain upon pressing (pressing pain) on the UB17 point (on the back, 1.5 cun from under the seventh cerebra).
   - Tongue index on the side of the tongue
   - Pressing pain on the SP10 point
   - Pressing pain on the SP6 point (mostly for bleeding in the lower abdomen)
   - Patient is thirsty but has no desire to drink water

Heart Disease

Myocardial Infarction and Angina Pectoris[4]

1. Use acupuncture on the REN14 point, under the eleventh vertebra, and on the ST45 point.
2. Use acupuncture on the SP4, PC6, REN14, and REN4 points.
3. If the pain is as sharp as a needle punching, use acupuncture on the REN14, UB15, HT7, PC8, HT8, and REN4 points.
4. Use acupuncture on the HT1 and REN17 points (especially for a feeling of pressure in the chest).
5. Use acupuncture on the PC6 point (especially for tachycardia or bradyarrhythmia).
6. Use acupuncture on the Coronary point.
7. Use acupuncture on the LU2 point.
8. Use acupuncture on the Chest-pain point.
9. Use folk therapy. Materials: one green onion, two fresh ginger, and two white turnips. Chop all material into mud. Bring to a warm temperature. Fold into gauze to paste on the painful area.

---

[4]. There could be pain on the tips of the middle fingers.

Heart Failure—When the Heart Is About to Stop Beating

1. Use acupuncture on the REN4 point and then the REN22 and REN14 points. The heart will start to beat again.

If the heart stops beating for less than half an hour (the left front chest is still warm), use the following treatment:

1. Use acupuncture on the DU26 point.
2. Use acupuncture on the REN4 and HT8 points.
3. Use UB35 nine needles.[5]
4. Give the herbal tea Mahuang Tang through a stomach tube.

    This may bring back consciousness for about another half hour, allowing the patient to give final words.

Panic Attack

1. Use acupuncture on the DU26 and DU20 points.
2. Use acupuncture on the REN15 and DU20 points.
3. Use acupuncture on the SJ1 point.
4. Use acupuncture on the KID1 point.
5. Use moxibustion on the HT7 and KID6 points.
6. Use acupuncture on the Shoulder-back point.

Epilepsy

1. Use bleeding therapy on the veins on the back of the ears.
2. Use acupuncture on the DU26 point.
3. Use acupuncture on the DU8 point (after the ninth vertebra) and the Yaoqi point.
4. Use acupuncture on the DU20 and KID1 points.

---

5. The needle inserts in nine directions around the point.

5. Use acupuncture on the REN15, DU26, KID1, and REN17 points.
6. Use acupuncture on the ST40 points.
7. Use acupuncture on the Shoulder-back point.

Hysteria

1. Use acupuncture on the DU26 point.
2. Use acupuncture on the DU20 and KID1 points (especially for hysteric paralysis).
3. Use acupuncture on the REN15 and DU20 points.
4. Use moxibustion on the HT7 and KID6 points.
5. Use acupuncture on the Shoulder-back point.
6. Use acupuncture with the thirteen-ghost-needle technique. This technique is for the treatment of a condition in which a spirit (ghost) resides inside the body of the patient. In such cases, the patient may speak like a different person by age and by sex. When using this technique, do the following:
   - Feel the pulse on the root side of the patient's middle fingers. If no pulse can be felt,[6] there is no need to use this technique.
   - Use acupuncture on points in this sequence: DU26, LU11, SP1, PC7, HT7, DU16, ST6, REN24, PC8, DU23, REN1, and Under-the-tongue points.
   - If the symptoms subside, there is no need to finish all the points.
   - If the patient speaks, ask what the patient wants (it is actually not the patient, but the spirit speaks). Try to meet its need and convince the spirit to leave.
   - If the doctor has no confidence to involve himself into such special treatment, do not use this technique.

---

6. The pulse here indicates the presence of a spirit inside the body of the patient.

Gynecology and Obstetrics
Bleeding from the Uterus
Ordinary Uterus Bleeding

1. Use acupuncture on the Shangdu point.
2. Use moxibustion on the SP1 point and then acupuncture on the Fuling point.

Uterus Bleeding after Birth Delivery

1. Use acupuncture on the SP1 point.
2. Use acupuncture on the LI4 and SP6 points.
3. Use acupuncture on the SJ6 and SP6 points.
4. Use acupuncture on the LI4, SP6, DU26, and ST36 points, and use moxibustion on the SP1 and REN4 points.
5. Use folk therapy.
   - Use 15 g hot pepper roots and four chicken's feet. Add the pepper roots and chicken's feet to water. Bring to a boil for twenty to thirty min. Drink the soup twice a day. After bleeding stops, the drink should still be consumed for five to ten days.
   - Burn one old luffa until dark in color. Grind into powder. Drink it with salt water, nine g each time, three times a day.
   - Cook 30 g of litchi in water for 5 min. Drink it as a tea every day. Continue for 15 days.

Dysmenorrhea

1. Use acupuncture on the point under the seventeenth vertebra.
2. Use acupuncture on the LIV5 and GB26 points.
3. Use acupuncture on the UB55 point.

4. Use acupuncture on the SP6, Linggu, and Menjin points.
5. Use folk therapy.

    - For lower stomach pain due to menstruation, use 15 g fresh ginger and 30 g brown sugar. Add the material to water. Bring to a boil for 30 min. Drink the soup.
    - For stomach pain due to menstruation, use 10 g Chinese prickly ash peel and 3 g pepper. Grind the material into a powder. Mix with liquor to prepare a paste. Apply the paste on the navel. Seal it with medical tape. Repeat every day. This tip works if the pain is due to the accumulation of cold in the lower stomach area (uterus).
    - For lower stomach pain before menstruation, add 15 g fennel to water. Bring to a boil for 30 min. Drink the extract every day, three days before the period begins.
    - For lower stomach pain before menstruation, use 500 ml liquor and 60 g salvia. Add the salvia to the liquor. Keep for one month. Drink the mixture several days before the period begins. This tip is mostly useful if the pain is caused by "blood stagnation" in the lower stomach.
    - For stomach pain before or during menstruation, cut dried luffa into small pieces. Add it to water. Bring to a boil for 30 to 60 min. Drink the extract. Repeat twice a day.
    - For lower back pain in women, add 30 g of luffa net material to water. Bring to a boil for 30 to 60 min. Drink the water extract together with a little cooking wine.

Fetus Malposition

1. Use acupuncture on the UB67 point.
2. Use moxibustion (direct or indirect) on the UB67, SP1, SP6, and GB25 points, 15 to 20 min each time, once a day for four days. For direct moxi, perform four to 5 cones each time.

    Note:

1. The success rate is highest with horizontal position, followed by hip position. The feet position is difficult.
2. The correction of the position occurs within four sessions.

Expedite Fetus Delivery
1. Use acupuncture on the LI4, SP6, and UB67 points.
2. Have the patient drink herbal Fupengzi (覆盆子) tea.

Note: It is reported that after acupuncture treatment, 38.1 percent of women started labor within twelve to twenty-four hours, and 32.7 percent started within twenty-four to forty-eight hours.

Retained Placenta
1. Use acupuncture on the UB67 point.
2. Use acupuncture on the SP6 and Duyin points, plus the REN4 or REN3 points.
3. Use acupuncture on the REN3, KID6, GB21, and SJ5 points.

Nocturnal Fretfulness in Infants
1. Use acupuncture on the PC9 point.
2. Use acupuncture on the DU20, PC6, SP6, HT7, and LIV2 points.
3. If there is a fever, use acupuncture on the LI4, PC6, Sifeng, PC9, and HT5 points.
4. If there are cold signs (face is pale, hands and feet are cold), use acupuncture on the DU20, Yintang, LI4, PC6, Sifeng, SP6, ST36, and REN10 points.
5. Use moxibustion on the DU20 and PC9 points.

Note:

1. For acupuncture in children, the acupuncture needle does not remain in the skin after there is acupuncture sensation (by the acupuncturist).
2. On the Sifeng point, stab the points (four points on each hand) with a lancet, and press out blood or white-colored liquid.

Burns (Fire, Boiling Water, and Similar)

1. Use bleeding therapy on the LU11 point.
2. Use acupuncture on local skin (in the middle and around the skin lesion) and then on the UB12, UB13, SP10, KID9, and SJ5 points.
3. Use herbal tea: Guizhi Tang (without the herb Shaoyao but with Shuti, Longgu, and Muli in the formula).
4. Smear on an herbal oil of Muli, the herb Daihuang, and Liuhuang, all ground into powder and mixed with sesame oil. If there are blisters on the skin, burn the herb Shichangpu into ash, and mix the ash in the oil lotion above to use.
5. Use folk therapy.

    - Use 30 g beeswax and 280 ml bean oil. Mix the wax and oil and melt. Clear the wound, and smear the paste on the affected skin. If there is no bean oil, simply smear clear honey on the affected skin.
    - Smear soy sauce on the affected skin before you can find some other way for healing.
    - Use soda diluted with six fold of water. Wash the skin (not broken skin) with the soda water.
    - Use thirty g of white sugar and three g of borneol (Bing Pian). Grind the material into powder. Mix with sesame oil to make a paste. Apply it to the burned skin.
    - Mix liquor and wheat powder to prepare a paste. Apply the paste on the affected skin. Change it whenever the paste becomes dry.

- Put old cucumber pulp into a bottle. Keep it in soil three feet deep for one week. Smear the juice in the bottle on the affected skin.
- Use old cucumber juice (pulp removed before the juice is made). Grind the cucumber into juice. Smear the juice on the affected skin.
- Smear pumpkin juice on the affected skin.
- Smear pumpkin cane juice on the affected skin.
- Bake wax gourd peel until yellow in color. Grind it into powder. Mix with a little sesame oil. Smear it on the affected skin.
- For scalds, use 100 g of banana. Grind it into mud. Apply to the affected skin twice a day.

Frostbite

1. Put the frostbitten skin in warm water, 38°C–42°C, until the skin color becomes red. It needs about 30 to 60 min. Do not use snow to rub or to warm it by a fire.
2. Wash the frostbitten skin with warmed ginger or hot pepper water. Cook the ginger or pepper in water for 20 to 30 min before use.
3. Use acupuncture on surrounding acupuncture points, whichever they are. Perform acupuncture around the affected skin, 0.2 centimeters from the edge of the lesion; quickly stab and take off the needle (do not retain the needle). Then perform acupuncture with several needles on the edge of the skin lesion and around the lesion, with intervals of 0.2–0.5 centimeters and a shallow stab. Again, use several needles around the lesion, and, in the lesion area, stab the needle with intervals of 0.25–0.5 centimeters. Repeat the inner acupuncture in circles until up to the center of the skin lesion (fewer and fewer needles in each circle). Finally, use one thick needle to stab bleeding (no needle retention). This acupuncture technique is used once every other day.

4. Use acupuncture on the SJ5, KID9, LI4, SJ3, and Baxie (for frostbite on the hands) points. Or LIV3, LIV2, ST41, UB60, and ST44 (for frostbite on the feet), or acupuncture points on the back of the ear (for frostbite on the ear). Choose three or four points each time; retain the needle for 30 min. Local bleeding therapy can be used together with acupuncture.

5. Use direct moxibustion on the skin lesion. Use a burned moxi roll. Quickly (two to three times per second) touch the frostbitten skin and lift. The frostbitten skin will feel slight burning pain, but there will be no scar later. Repeat this for 5 to 10 min once a day or once every other day, with seven sessions as one healing period.

6. Use indirect moxibustion on frostbitten skin. Put a thin piece of fresh ginger (about two millimeters thick and two to three centimeters in diameter) on the skin. Put a moxi cone (about one centimeter high and one centimeter in diameter) on it. Burn the moxi cone. Move it aside after the patient feels a strong burning sensation (do not leave the skin), until the moxi no longer gives a burning sensation. Repeat three to five such cone burnings for each session, once a day, for five days.

7. Use bleeding therapy on the frostbitten skin. Use a triangle-edged needle to make the frostbitten skin bleed. The amount of blood is about 0.2–0.3 ml each time and once a day. If the intensity of the frozen damage is very heavy, additional herbal therapy should be also considered.

8. Use folk therapy.

    - Combine four parts honey with one part pig oil. Melt the honey and oil, and prepare into a paste. Smear it on the affected skin, once in the morning and once in the afternoon.

    - Apply warm vinegar on the frostbitten skin. Repeat several times a day.

    - Use 30 ml liquor, 15 g Chinese prickly ash peel, 3 ml fresh ginger juice, and 6 ml glycerin. Add the ash peel to the liquor, and keep it for one week. Remove the peel. Add the ginger juice and glycerin, and mix well. Smear it on the affected skin.

- Add cabbage to water. Bring to a boil for 30 to 60 min. Wash the frostbitten skin with the water extract every night before going to bed.
- Add eggplant stems and roots to water. Bring to a boil for 10 to 20 min. Wash hands and feet with the water every night before going to bed. Or you can add eggplant root and Chinese prickly ash (Hua Jiao) to water. Bring to a boil for 10 to 20 min. Wash hands and feet with the water every night before going to bed. It is used for frostbite without broken skin.

Note:

If the skin is broken, smear Yunnan Baoyao[7] powder on the wound. Fold with gauze, and fix it with tape.

Herbal formula used as oral therapy for frostbite: 6 g Guizhi, 12 g Baishao, 10 g Danggui, three pieces fresh ginger, 10 g Chinese red date, and 5 g Zhi Gancai. Cook in 1000 ml of water, and collect 600 ml to drink (300 ml each time). This is a one-day dose.

Herbal formula used as oral therapy for frostbite: 10 g Danggui, 10 g Guizhi, 10 g Baishao, 3 g Xixin, 5 g Gancao, 6 g Mutong, 3 g Wuzhuyu, and 9 g fresh ginger. Cook in 1000 ml water, and collect 600 ml to drink (300 ml each time). This is a one-day dose.

Drowning

1. Remove the clothes from the person's body. Put the person face down, lift the lower back higher but keep the chest lower, and press the chest to allow the water out.

---

7. *Yunnan* is the name of a province in China. *Bai* means "white color" and *yao* means "herbs" in Chinese.

2. Cardiorespiratory resuscitation is commonly used in Western medicine. This is the standard way by conventional medicine to save the life of a drowning person. It may work within a half hour after the heartbeat stops.

Chinese medicine has its own way for such an emergency:

1. Perform procedure one above.
2. Clean the ear, navel, mouth, and nose. Open the mouth, pull out the tongue, and use a chopstick (or similar thing) to put in the mouth in a horizontal manner (two ends of the stick are out of the mouth) to keep the mouth open. Blow air into both ears (by two doctors) with the mouth directly or with a tube (any kind of tube).
3. Pour liquor into the nose. Or blow herbal powder (Xixin and Banxia, equal amounts) or hot pepper powder into the nostrils. Or pour fresh duck blood into the mouth.
4. Blow herbal Zaojiao (saponin) powder or Duanshi (lime) powder into the anus.
5. Smear cooking salt on the navel, and use moxibustion on the navel (or without salt, but do not touch the navel with burning moxi). Stab the Shixuan points.
6. At the same time, perform acupuncture on the DU26, DU25, PC6, ST36, and KID1 points. Use bleeding therapy on the PC9 point (with a triangle-edged needle).
7. You can also perform acupuncture on the SP4, PC6, and REN12 points. Then turn the body face down, bend the patient's knee, and perform acupuncture on the REN1 point (figure 8). After the patient wakes up, and if the body temperature is still low, have the patient drink the herbal tea Ganjiang Fuzi Tang.

You can also do the following:
1. Use acupuncture on the LI4, LIV3, DU26, and DU1 points. Open the person's mouth, pull out the tongue, fix it with a chopstick (or something similar) to prevent

the tongue slipping back to block the trachea, and blow air into both ears with a hollow tube (or with the doctor's mouth directly).

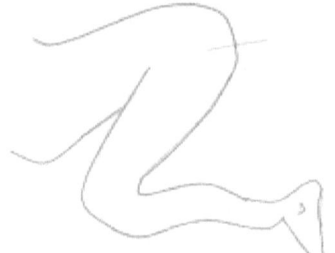

Figure 8. Body position when punctured on REN1 point

2. Let a strong man hold the feet of the drowned person on his shoulder, with the patient's back against the man's back. Let the head of the person be down. Let the man run for 10 to 30 min.
3. Put the body of the drowned person on the back of a cow or a horse (face down), and let the cow or horse walk. Or put the drowned person's body face down over a normal person (the normal person is face up), navel to navel, shaking the body of the normal person continuously.
4. Bury the drowned person's body with grass ash[8] or soil collected from a soil wall,[9] leaving the mouth, nose, ears, and anus open. The ash or soil should be changed if it becomes wet. (The usefulness of this technique can be tested with a drowned fly or small animals, such as a rat or a bird.)

All of the above procedures can be performed, whichever is available.

Note:

---

8. Do not use the ash from the burning of coal.
9. Scratch the soil from the side of the wall that faces the sun during daytime.

1. With modern techniques, for those who have been drowning for more than twenty-five min, the death rate is 100 percent. According to Chinese medicine, even if the person is "dead" for up to twenty-four hours due to drowning, the life can still be saved.
2. Upon acupuncture on the REN1 point, if stool or urine comes out, it suggests that the person can be saved.
3. The REN1 point can be stabbed with a triangle-edged needle. Cover the needle tip with a thin layer of soap before use. If the person usually has constipation, it is not easy to allow the stool to come out. In this case, insert a piece of soap in and out of the anus several times to stimulate the stool to come out.
4. In most cases, drowning happens suddenly, and it is outdoors. But a lifeguard working at a swimming pool or beach should be able to keep the herbal powder on hand in case it is needed.
5. Any of the regularly used moxibustion treatments can be used, such as direct moxi or indirect moxi with fresh ginger over the acupuncture points (on the REN6, REN4, and UB23 points). This can speed up first aid.
6. Warm up the chest first (for example, use a hot water bag folded with several layers of towel). Do not warm up the body by letting it directly face a fire.
7. The success rate is higher in summer than in winter.
8. It has been indicated in Chinese literature from history that the Chinese ways can save the life of a drowned person who has lost heartbeat and has stopped breathing for more than twenty-four hours.
9. The Chinese way of saving a life from drowning introduced here could be a very big question and unbelievable from a conventional medicine point of view.[10] It is recommended that the doctor can still use the

---

10. Considering that a drowned person can be saved in such a way, the author strongly suspects that the life of a "dead" person can still be saved, even if the lack

conventional medicine ways first. If the person has been declared to be "dead" after trying the conventional ways, why not try the Chinese way also?

Heatstroke

1. Use acupuncture on the DU26, Shixuan, and LU11 points.
2. Use acupuncture on the PC6, LI4, and ST36 points.
3. If there is a coma, use acupuncture on the DU26 and DU25 points.
4. Use acupuncture on the shoulder-pain one point.
5. Use folk therapy.

    - Bean soup: 10 g soya bean, 10 g black soya bean, and 10 g mung bean. All are cooked in 300 ml water until the

---

of heartbeat and breathing has lasted for hours—providing that the reason for the stopping of heartbeat and breathing is sudden and due to some special reasons, such as a big blast (as in a war or on a construction site), a scare in a big fire (no severe burning damage to the body), a scare in an accident, a scare by thunder, a scare by sudden extremely good news, and so on. It means that the reason for the arrest of heartbeat and breathing is sudden, not the end result of a severe disease. This hypothesis may well explain the frequent story about how a soldier woke up several hours after his fellow soldiers left him on the field because they believed that he was dead. Presumably, his comrades had tested his heartbeat and breathing before they concluded that he was dead. People may argue that the solder might still have a heartbeat, although it could not be felt on the artery on the neck. The fact is that if the pulse cannot be felt on the artery in the neck or on the chest, blood pressure must be very low. According to conventional medicine, an insufficient supply of blood due to low blood pressure will soon result in kidney and liver failure. So the saving of life later should not be possible. But such cases happen again and again. It can even happen in a morgue where a patient wakes up there by himself after the doctor checked his ECG before declaring his death. However, considering there are different reasons for the sudden stopping of heartbeat and breathing, the way to save a life could be different from the ways we used here for a drowned person. For example, if the reason is due to a fire or a thunder attack (both belong to fire damage), moxibustion (fire) should not be used; the body should be kept in water (water is against fire) or buried with soil that is collected from a soil wall, the side of which is against the sun (the Yin side of the wall), and so on. I present the discussion in more detail here because saving a life is the most urgent challenge in the emergency department.

beans are soft and edible. Drink the soup, and eat the beans. Everyone can drink this soup in hot summer.
- Pear plus crystal sugar. Chop the pear into pieces, and grind the crystal sugar into powder. Eat both.
- Combine five to eight plums and two teaspoons white sugar. Cook in water until the plums become soft. Drink the soup as a regular beverage.

Note:
1. Move the person to a colder, fresh air environment.
2. If there is a coma or shock, treat the conditions in the ways described for those conditions.

Carbon Monoxide Toxicity

1. Use acupuncture on the DU26, DU25, KID1, and Shixuan points (bleeding therapy from the Shixuan points).
2. If the patient is vomiting, use acupuncture on the PC6 and ST36 points.
3. If the patient has an annoyed feeling and pressure feeling on chest, use acupuncture on the REN17 and REN12 points.
4. Use moxibustion on the DU20, REN8, and REN6 points.
5. Use folk therapy.
   - Mix one cup of tea (high concentration) and one cup vinegar. Drink it throughout the day.
   - Mix well 500 ml white radish juice with honey. Drink it.
   - For life-threatening toxins, such as arsenic, strong acid or alkaline, and others, let the person drink strong green tea (high-concentration tea) before and during transporting the person to the emergency department. The tea neutralizes the toxin and partially moves the toxin through the urine.

Note:

1. Move the person to a fresh air environment.
2. If there is a coma or shock, treat the conditions in the ways introduced in the corresponding chapters.

Acute and Heavy Dizziness

1. Use acupuncture on the GB20, Taiyang, UB18, UB23, LIV3, and KID3 points.
2. Use acupuncture on the DU20 point.
3. Use acupuncture on the SJ1 point.
4. Use acupuncture on the Shoulder-pain one point.

Note:
1. It is better to establish the diagnosis for the dizziness according to Chinese medicine.
2. It is better to use Chinese herbal therapy.

Acute Pain on the Body's Surface
Migraine

1. Use bleeding therapy on the veins on the back of the ear.
2. Use acupuncture on the DU4 point.
3. Use acupuncture on the LI4 point (on the healthy side) and Taiyang point (on the sick side, penetrating to the GB8 point).
4. Use acupuncture on the GB8 point.
5. Use acupuncture on the Shoulder-pain one point.
6. If there is nausea or vomiting, use acupuncture on the REN12, PC6, ST36, or SP4 points.
7. Use acupuncture on the REN12 point (for pain on the front of the head), UB67 point (for pain on the back of the head), or LIV3 point (pain on the side of the head).
8. Use folk therapy.

- Add ten stems of hot pepper roots to water, and bring to a boil for 10 to 20 min. Mix with a little bit of brown sugar to drink.
- Wash celery roots, and chop them into small pieces. Fry them with chicken eggs. Eat the eggs twice a day.
- Mix white radish juice with a little borneol (Bing Pian). Drip the mixture into the nose. Drip in the right nostril if the pain is on the left side; drip in the left nostril if the pain is on the right side.
- For a person with a headache, it is easy to experience blurred vision. Wash 30 to 60 g of banana skin clean, add to water, and cook as a soup. Drink as a green tea every day.
- Cook 15 g litchi, 12 g Gamdir Vine, 12 g Ur (Gou Ten), and 9 g rock sugar in water for 30 min. Drink the soup twice a day after a meal.
- For headache due to hypertension, mix 50 g peach branch and 12 g cassia seed (Jue ming zi). Add to water, and cook as a soup. Drink the extract twice a day.

Trigeminal Neuralgia

1. Use acupuncture on the LI4 point.
2. Use acupuncture on the GB8 point.
3. Use acupuncture on the Yuyao, ST2, and ST7 points.
4. Use acupuncture on the Taiyang, GB20, ST7, ST6, and LI4 points.

Bell's Palsy

1. Use acupuncture on the ST4 point (penetrating to the ST6 point). Treat the healthy side first, and then treat the sick side the next day.
2. Use acupuncture on the SI18 and ST7 points.

3. Use acupuncture on the ST6 point.
4. Smear eel blood on the sick face.

Headache Due to High Blood Pressure

The blood pressure is high. The face is red in color.

1. Use acupuncture on the ST36-xia[11] point (one cun distance below the ST36 point). The needle tip is toward the ST36 point to guide the body Qi falling down.
2. Use acupuncture on the LI11 point.
3. Use acupuncture on the GB8 point.
4. Use acupuncture on the REN12 point (mostly for front headache).
5. Use acupuncture on the LIV3 point (mostly for side headache).
6. Use acupuncture on the UB67 point (mostly for back head pain).
7. Use acupuncture on the Shoulder-pain one point.

Neck Stiffness

1. Have the patient lie on a bed with the head falling off the edge of the bed and keep the posture for several min. Crawl up with the person's own hands and feet back to the bed (to move the head back on the bed) (figure 9).
2. Use acupuncture on the SI3 and HT7 points. If this does not work, use acupuncture on the GB21 and ST36 points.
3. Use acupuncture on the UB10, UB11, and GB20 points.
4. Use acupuncture on the LI10 and GB39 points.
5. Use acupuncture on the SJ3 point.
6. Use acupuncture on the Shoulder-pain two point.

---

11. *Xia* means "below" in Chinese.

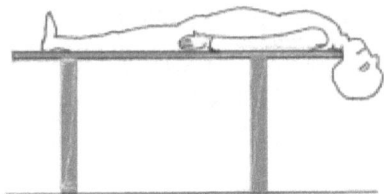

Figure 9. Body posture when having neck stiffness. Crawl up onto the bed with hands and feet.

Acute Shoulder Pain

1. Use acupuncture on the Shoulder-pain two point.

2. Use acupuncture on the Shoulder-pain one point.

3. Use acupuncture on the ST38 point (deep to penetrating to the UB57 point).

4. Use acupuncture on the Jianqi point.

5. Use acupuncture on the Shoulder-back point (two cun away from the tailbone).

6. Use acupuncture on the HT7 point, plus one of the following points: LI2 (if the pain is worse when the person stretches the arm out), SI3 (if the person feels more pain when bending the arm back to touch the shoulder blade), or SJ3 (if the person feels more pain when touching the head).

7. Ask the person to lift the arm (shoulder) to let the pain come out and keep the posture. Use acupuncture on the pain spot, with the needle along the muscle fiber direction, about 2.5 cun in depth. Ask the person to move the shoulder 50 times. If this spot has no more pain, but there is a new spot, do acupuncture the same way. Then ask the person to lie on the side with the sick shoulder up. Puncture the LI15 point. Keep the needle in place for 30 min. Use cupping on the painful spot.

8. Use acupuncture on the SI9, SJ14, and LI15 points, plus the Ashi point, with one or two of the following points: GB21, SI11, LI10, or LI11.

9. Use bleeding therapy plus cupping. On the LU5, LI11, or PC3 points, choose clear veins, and use the triangle-edged needle to leak out about 5 to 10 ml of dark blood. Do cupping on the point for 5 min. Repeat the bleeding and cupping after ten days.

10. Use acupuncture on the Jianjiahui point. For males, the point is 0.5 cun above the root of the penis. For females, it is the lower edge of the synchondroses pubis. Use light stimulation.

11. Use acupuncture on the SI11 point. (Stab the SI11 point first, lift the needle up under the skin, turn the needle tip toward the DU14 point, and then lift the needle under the skin and turn to the shoulder direction.) Then use acupuncture on the SJ3 and ST38 points.

Acute Pain on the Elbow

1. Use acupuncture on the SP9 point.
2. Use acupuncture on the ST42 point (on the sick side).
3. Use acupuncture on the HT3, LI12, and LU5 points.
4. Use acupuncture on the ST35 point.
5. Use acupuncture on the LI20 and LI1 points.
6. Use acupuncture on the LI10, LI2, and LI3 points.
7. Use acupuncture on the pressing pain point on the inner side of the knee (on healthy knee).
8. Use acupuncture on the Sizhi[12] point (one and one-half cun under the SP9 point).
9. Use acupuncture on the GB41, GB34, ST44, ST37, UB57, or UB23 points.
10. Use acupuncture on the LI11, LI12, LI10, LI13, and Ashi points with one or two of the following points: LI8 (if the pain is worse when the front arm turns inward), LU5 (if the pain is worse when the front arm turns outward), HT3 (if the

---

12. *Si* means "four"; *zhi* means "arms or legs" in Chinese.

pain is more inside the elbow), or SJ10 (if the pain is more on the back of the elbow). For the Ashi point (the painful spot), the needle can be stabbed in multiple directions, or you can use more needles around the point.

11. Use a fire needle on the Ashi point. It can be repeated after three or five days.
12. Use bleeding-and-cupping therapy on the Ashi point around the elbow.
13. Use bleeding-and-cupping therapy on points between the ST36 and ST40 points on the same side of the leg.

Acute Wrist Pain

1. Use acupuncture on the KID3 point.
2. Use acupuncture on the SJ5 point.
3. Use acupuncture on the hand's low-back-pain points (two points on the back of the hand).
4. Use acupuncture on the PC7 point (needle tip is toward the middle finger), plus the following points: LU8 and LU6 (if there is numbness in thumb), LI5 and LI4 (if there is numbness in the point finger), PC6 (penetrating to SJ5) and Zhongbai and Xiabai (if there is numbness in the middle finger), SJ3 and DU15 (if there is swelling and redness on the back of the hand), HT7 and SP6 (if there is poor sleep), or LU10 (if there is a muscle withered in the thumb).
5. Use acupuncture on the SI3 point (penetrating to PC8) for hand numbness.
6. Use acupuncture on the Baxie point for finger pain and numbness.
7. Use acupuncture on the SI6 point.

Acute Back Pain

1. Use acupuncture on the DU20 point (sitting posture).

2. Use acupuncture on the DU26, UB40, and GB34 points (if the pain is mostly on the middle of the spine, and if the pain occurs for less than forty-eight hours).
3. Use acupuncture on the head's low-back-pain point (if the pain is on the side of the spine). It is located in the middle of the front of the head.
4. Use acupuncture on the hand's low-back-pain point (if the pain is on the side of the spine). It is located on the back of the hand, with two spots on each hand.
5. Use acupuncture on the UB23, GB30, UB57, SI3, and DU26 points.
6. Use acupuncture on the thunder-flash point. Let the person stand facing the bed, with hands holding the bed and the upper body slightly bending to the front, both legs standing lengthwise. Stab the needle with a strong twist or pulling-inserting. After the person gets the feeling of electric shock up or down the leg, take off the needle. Let the person move the back slowly after the acupuncture.
7. Use acupuncture on the SJ3 and LI10 points.
8. Use acupuncture on the UB40, LI10, and UB58 points.
9. Use acupuncture on the UB40, GB30, and SI3 points.
10. Use acupuncture on the UB40 and the head's low-back-pain points.
11. Use acupuncture on the UB40 and DU8 points (especially for protrusion of lumbar intervertebral disc).
12. Use acupuncture on the Shoulder-pain two point, as deep as two cun.
13. Use acupuncture on the Hip-pain point.
14. Use acupuncture on the LI10, UB57, and KID7 points.
15. Use acupuncture on the LI4 and PC7 points (for pain on hips).
16. Use acupuncture on the SI6 point.
17. Use acupuncture on the Shangdu point.

18. Use acupuncture on the Spine point (between the SI2 and SI3 points).
19. Use the Tuina technique. Massage the bruise point (middle point between the UB57 point and the bottom of the heel). Use the same side. Massage the pain spot on the back and the horizontally reflecting point on the abdomen (massage the two points at the same time when the person exhales).
20. Use bleeding-and-cupping therapy on the painful spot and the UB40 point.
21. Use folk therapy. Press 60 g Chinese chives to collect juice. Mix the juice with 60 ml cooking wine. Drink it three times a day.

Note:
1. For most of the acupuncture treatment, the patient can be either in a standing posture or sitting down.
2. If the pain is in the middle line of the spine, it's better not to use massage techniques.
3. The above acupuncture groups can be combined.
4. For acute pain, the stimulation is strong and the needle is not needed to be kept for longer than several min.
5. Whenever possible, ask the person to slightly move the lower back during and after the acupuncture treatment.

Acute Sciatic Pain
1. Use acupuncture on the LI4 point.
2. Use acupuncture on the Hip-pain point.
3. Use acupuncture on the SI3 point.
4. Use acupuncture on the SJ3 point.
5. Use acupuncture on the Shoulder-pain one point.
6. Use acupuncture on the Shoulder-back point.

7. Use acupuncture on the GB30, GB34, UB37, UB40, UB57, and UB60 points (for the pain distributed along the Taiyang meridian).
8. Use acupuncture on the GB30, GB34, GB31, GB33, GB38, and GB39 points (for pain distributed along the Shaoyang meridian).
9. Use acupuncture on the GB30, GB34, and Huanzhongshang points (bend the thigh, two cun over the middle point between the tailbone and the trochiter), plus one or two of the following points: UB40, UB23, Baliao,[13] UB60, UB37, and GB40.
10. Use acupuncture on the UB1 and UB67 points (for pain along the Taiyang meridian), the GB1 and GB44 points (for pain along the Shaoyang meridian), the UB1 and SI19 points, or the UB2 and GB20 points. Two points in each group should be inserted at the same time (by two operators). For the UB1 point, press the eyeball outside, and then insert the needle with no pulling or inserting after insertion of the needle.

Note:
1. The stem-type sciatic pain is usually caused by lumbar disc protrusion. The pain is from the lower back to the feet.
2. The branch-type sciatic pain is mostly along the distribution zone of the sciatic nerve.
3. For the treatment of sciatic pain, it is better to use electric acupuncture.

Acute Tailbone Pain

1. Use acupuncture on the DU20 and DU19 points.
2. Use acupuncture on the Shoulder-back point.

---

13. Baliao: UB31, UB32, UB33, and UB34 on both sides.

3. Use acupuncture on the Baliao point.
4. Use acupuncture on the UB25, Baliao, UB54, and UB60 points.
5. Use acupuncture on the DU1, Yaoqi, DU2, DU3, UB40, and LI4 points.
6. Use bleeding therapy on the UB57 point.

Acute Knee Pain

1. Use acupuncture on the UB11 and LI11 points.
2. Use acupuncture on the PC6 and LIV8 points.
3. Use acupuncture on the inner-Xiyan and outer-Xiyan points.
4. Use acupuncture on the Bingu, ST34 (needle toward the feet), SP10 (needle toward the feet), and ST35 points.
5. Use acupuncture on the Linggu, Dabai, and Jianzhong points (needle toward the knee for the Jianzhong point).
6. Use acupuncture on the LI11, LU5, SI8, and SJ10 points.
7. Use acupuncture on the Kuangu and Xiguan points (one cun back from the SP9 point).
8. Use acupuncture on the tender spot on the lower abdomen (mostly on the sick knee side).
9. Use acupuncture on the Xiguan, UB40, and ST36 points.
10. Do point pressing on the Xiaogukong point with a bead. (Put a bead on a medical tape, stick the tape on the acupuncture point with the bead toward the point, and press the bead from time to time.) The point is located on the back of the small finger, the middle of the joint between the base stem and the middle stem of the small finger (figure 21).
11. Use bleeding-and-cupping therapy on the UB43 point on the back.
12. Use bleeding-and-cupping therapy on the painful spots or the spots with clear veins on the knee.

13. Use bleeding-and-cupping therapy on the UB40 point of the sick knee.
14. Use folk therapy. Add 3 g cinnamon and 9 g fresh ginger to water. Bring to a boil for 30 min. Drink the extract.

Calf Spasm
1. Use acupuncture on the UB57 point (deep into the bone).
2. Use acupuncture on the GB34 point.
3. Have the patient drink warm sucrose water.

Note:
1. Upon the spasm, pull the big toe toward the direction of the back of the foot. The heel pushes down and stretches the knee to even.
2. Stretch the arm of the opposite side. For example, if the left calf is in spasm, lift and stretch the right arm up.
3. Press the DU26 point.
4. Press the inner side of the knee; you can feel a hard muscle and tendon. Press this tendon (it is the attaching point of the calf to the inner side of the knee).
5. Massage the UB40 point (back of the knee), and then move down to the heel.
6. Press the UB57 point (back of the calf) with both thumbs for 2 min. Tap the calf muscle.

Acute Bruise on the Ankle
1. Use acupuncture on the GB40 (penetrating to the SP5 point), SJ5, and ST41 points.
2. Use acupuncture on the ST41 and PC7 points.
3. Use acupuncture on the LI4 point.
4. Use acupuncture on the SP21 point (for bruises anywhere).

5. Use acupuncture on the GB39, SP6, UB60, and ST41 points and on the painful spot.
6. Use acupuncture on the GB40, HT7, UB60, GB39, and GB34 points (mostly for outside pain) or the SP5, KID6, KID3, SP6, and SP9 points (mostly for inner side pain).
7. Use folk therapy.

    - Chop the leaves of green onions into a mud/paste. Apply to the affected joints.
    - If the skin is not broken, you can smear vinegar on the skin to reduce swelling and pain.
    - Materials: 60 ml liquor, 9 g camphor, and several drops fresh ginger juice. Add the camphor into the liquor to dissolve. Add several drops of fresh ginger, and mix it again. Smear the mixture on the affected skin three to five times a day.
    - Burn liquor. Apply the liquor (still under burn) to the joint.
    - Materials: 90 g Chinese chive roots and 30 g wheat powder. Chop the chive roots into mud. Mix with wheat powder to prepare into a paste. Add a little bit of liquor. Mix all, and apply the mixture to the affected joints.
    - Materials: 30 g Chinese chive leaves and some fresh ginger juice. Chop the chives into mud. Mix with the ginger juice. Apply the mixture to the affected joints.
    - Chop fresh Chinese chives with the addition of a little salt into mud. Apply the mud to the affected ankle. Change to fresh-prepared mud every day. Repeat for days.

Acute Pain on the Heel
1. Use acupuncture on the PC7 point.
2. Use acupuncture on the KID3 and KID7 points.
3. Use acupuncture on the LI4 point. With the needle in the point, ask the patient to stamp his or her foot.

4. Use acupuncture on the Jiangqi point. With the needle in the point, ask the patient to stamp his or her foot.
5. Use acupuncture on the SP6-Hou point.
6. Use acupuncture on the UB10 point.
7. Use acupuncture on the LI15 point (penetrating to the HT1 point).
8. Use moxibustion on the KID3 and UB60 points (indirect moxi with fresh ginger on the points).
9. Cook 120 g of the herb Baizhu in water. Have a footbath in the herbal water.
10. Cook 120 g of the herb Mugua and 10 g Niuxi in water. Have a footbath in the herbal water.
11. Grind 20 g of the herb Weilingxian into powder, mix with vinegar into a mud, and apply the mud to the pain spot (fold and fix with gauze and tape).
12. Grind 24 g of the herb Huajiao and 60 g of Ruxiang into powder, mix with vinegar and egg yolk into a mud, and apply the mud to the pain spot (fold and fix with gauze and tape).

Note: For the treatment of heel pain, usually one to two acupuncture points are sufficient.

Foot Pain
1. Use acupuncture on the Bafeng points.
2. Use acupuncture on the Shouqianjin and Shouwujin points.
3. Use acupuncture on the UB40, UB57, KID1, ST41, and UB25 points.
4. Use acupuncture on the GB40, SP5, ST41, and LIV2 points.
5. Perform acupuncture using the methods above for the treatment of heel pain.

Gout

1. Use acupuncture on the KID7 and KID9 points.
2. Use bleeding therapy for bleeding from the painful joint. (Find the blue veins. If there are no blue veins, use a lancet to start bleeding around the pain area.) Then use acupuncture on the DU20, DU24, LI11, LI4, HT7, ST36, LIV3, ST40, ST44, and SP9 points. The acupuncture is performed once a day. Five sessions are one healing period.
3. Use bleeding therapy as above, and then use acupuncture on the SP2, Taibai, ST44, ST43, SP6, and GB34 points. Retain the needles for 30 min.
4. Use triple-edge needle acupuncture on the Bafeng and Baxie points. Press out a little blood or slightly yellow liquid.

Note for all the pain syndromes on the muscles and tendons:

1. Acute pain means the pain occurred within forty-eight hours.
2. The acupuncture treatments listed here can be combined, but do not use more than two treatments at the same time.
3. The acupuncture can be combined with moxibustion or with bleeding therapy.
4. With the needle in the points, ask the person to move the painful part of the body if the movement does not increase the pain.
5. Choose the acupuncture on the opposite side of the pain spot first. For example, if the pain is on the right shoulder, choose the acupuncture points on the left leg first and then acupuncture points on the right shoulder or right arm.
6. If the typical treatments listed above do not work, the next step is to choose the equal spots on the opposite side of the body. For example, if the pain is on the right shoulder, choose the left shoulder. It's better to press the left shoulder to find a tender spot and stab the needle on that spot, which may or may not be an acupuncture point.

7. The location of the acupuncture point listed above is a reference location. You'll need to find the tender spot on and around the indicated point, which is called the "active acupuncture point."
8. If the acupuncture needle is not available, the points can be stimulated with finger pressure or with an electric machine such as the Haihua acupuncture machine, which puts a probe onto the skin. There are many brands of such machines on the market.
9. If the pain has been there for a long time, but this time is worse, and several types of treatment have been tried but did not work well, see if there are sticky fibers or tendons that need to be loosened with a small knife needle.
10. For acupuncture with needles, basically the needles can be connected with an electric acupuncture machine to stimulate the acupuncture points with electricity. The intensity is adjusted until the needle is slightly shaking. The stimulation should remain for 20 to 30 min.

Herpes Zoster

1. Use acupuncture on the herpes point.
2. Use acupuncture around the skin lesion and the Jiaji, SJ6, and GB34 points. If the skin lesion is in the upper body, add the LI11, LI4, and SJ5 points. If it is in the lower body, add the SP6, LIV3, and SP10 points.
3. Apply four to eight needles around the skin lesion in a declining way toward the center of the lesion (one to three centimeters beside the edge of the lesion). Choose the Jiaji points, the nerve under which distributes to the lesion skin zone. The needle remains for 5 to 10 min and is twisted from time to time. The acupuncture is once or twice a day.
4. Use fire-needle acupuncture on the UB13, UB19, UB20, and Ashi points, once every three days. It usually needs one to three times. For the Ashi point, use several needles around the skin lesion.

5. There are two ways of moxibustion. For the first, use a moxi pile (rice size) on the skin lesion, which is the first lesion, and on another lesion where there are a lot of clustered blisters. Burn it until the patient feels too hot. Blow off the moxi pile. Repeat this to another zone of the skin lesion once a day. If the lesion is not cured, repeat the moxibustion after five days. For the second way, burn a moxi roll (moving the roll above the skin lesion in a linear way along the long axis of the skin lesion or in a round circle from the edge to the center or from the center to the surrounding edge of the skin lesion), and warm the skin lesion for 30 min. This needs to be done once a day for four to seven days as a healing period.

6. Use fire-moxibustion on the PC6 and UB40 points or the LU7 and LI4 points. If the lesion is on the arms or legs, add the GB34 point. If the lesion is on the stomach, add the ST36 and SP6 points. If the lesion is on the hip, add the GB30 point. For this therapy, use a cotton wire. Dip it in sesame oil, burn it, and quickly touch it onto the acupuncture points. Once it touches the skin, lift it off. The skin spot may have a blister later. Leave it without special treatment. Do this therapy once a day, with four times as a healing period. The pain should subside within one to four days.

7. Perform flower-needle tapping on the skin along the spine (two centimeters from the middle line of the spine). If the skin lesion is on the chest, choose the length of the whole thoracic vertebra. If it is on the abdomen, choose the length of the whole lumbar vertebra. There is also tapping around the skin lesion (not touching the skin lesion). Tapping is three times on every line, once or twice a day.

8. Perform cupping on the skin lesion. The cup is retained for 15 min. If the blister is broken, use blister tape to cover it. This therapy is done once a day.

Acute Pain in the Mouth, Throat, or Abdomen

Toothache

1. Use acupuncture on the LI4 and ST7 points for upper teeth (on healthy side).
2. Use acupuncture on the LI4 and GB21 points.
3. Use acupuncture on the ST44 point for lower teeth (on healthy side).
4. Use acupuncture on the Low-back-pain point.
5. Use folk therapy.
   - Drop clove oil onto teeth.
   - For tooth decay, clear the filling of the tooth decay. Apply garlic mud.
   - Add six g Chinese prickly ash peel to 100 ml vinegar. Bring to a boil for 10 min. Remove the peel. Rinse mouth with the vinegar.
   - For continuous bleeding after tooth pulling, dissolve salt in water to prepare a high-concentration salt solution. Use a cotton ball to dip the salt solution. Apply the cotton to the bleeding area of the tooth. Take it away after one hour.
   - Mix 10 g Chinese chives and 20 grains prickly ash. Grind into powder. Mix the powder with a little sesame oil to prepare a paste. Smear the paste on the affected face skin.
   - Burn some apricot kernel into ash. Grind into powder. Apply into the hole of the dental caries.
   - Add one banana skin and 10 g rock sugar to water, and cook as a soup. Drink the soup twice a day.
   - Eat one peeled banana, dipping it into salt.

Mouth Ulcer

1. Use acupuncture as for a sore throat (see below).
2. Use folk therapy.

- Mix salt and sesame oil. Hold it in the mouth. For a baby, drop several drops in the mouth before feeding. Repeat several times a day.
- For mouth ulcer, gum ulcer, or tongue ulcer, rinse mouth with high-concentration tea. Repeat it from time to time for more than ten times a day.
- Choose a frost eggplant. Dry it naturally in the air. Grind it into powder. Smear it on the ulcer. You can also mix the powder with honey, and then smear it on the ulcer.
- Hold tomato juice in the mouth. Do this several times a day.
- Drink 100 g strawberry juice in the morning and at night.

Acute Pain in the Throat

1. Use acupuncture on the LU11, SJ1, and KID1 points.
2. Use acupuncture on the REN23 point.
3. Use acupuncture on the SJ3 point (especially for pain in tonsils).
4. Use folk therapy.

    - Grind garlic into a paste. Apply to the acupuncture point named Yu Ji (the big muscle close to the inside root of the thumb). Fold with gauze and medicine tape. After several hours, the skin will have a water blister. Protect the skin lesion with blister tape.
    - Add one part honey to eight parts hot water. Mix it well. Hold the honey water in the mouth. Do this several times every day.
    - Fry salt powder until warm. Blow it into the throat. The person will vomit out a lot of saliva. The pain will be reduced.
    - For frequent sore throats, drink salt water, 100 to 300 ml, every morning. Repeat every day for two to three weeks.

- Cut one frost luffa into small pieces. Add it to water, and bring it to a boil for 30 to 60 min. Drink the water extract.
- Chop one young luffa, and make it into juice. Drink the juice three times a day, 20 ml each time.
- Add fifty g loquat leaves and 25 g *Lophatherum gracile* Brongn (Dan Zhu Ye) to water to cook as a soup. Drink the soup as a tea from time to time. Repeat for several days.
- Drink 100 g strawberry juice in the morning and at night.

Acute Mumps

1. Use acupuncture as for a sore throat.
2. Use folk therapy.
   - Put gauze into vinegar. Take it out, and apply to the painful skin. Repeat several times a day.
   - Burn a luffa until it is black in color. Grind it into powder. Mix with chicken egg white. Smear on the affected skin.
   - Chop luffa leaves and stems to prepare juice. Smear the juice on the affected skin.
   - For tonsil inflammation, mix 60 ml white radish juice, 30 ml sugarcane juice, and some white sugar. Drink it three times a day.

Acute Gastritis

1. Use acupuncture on the ST36 and ST34 points.
2. Use acupuncture on the REN12, ST36, UB10, and PC6 points.
3. Use acupuncture on the PC6 and KID6 points.
4. Use acupuncture on the Yintang and Stomach-pain points.
5. Use acupuncture on the ST34 point.
6. Use acupuncture on the PC3 point.

7. Use acupuncture on the GB40 and REN13 points.
8. Use cupping on the UB20, UB21, REN12, and ST21 points.
9. Use folk therapy.
   - Materials: 30 g fresh ginger, one egg, and 30 ml sesame oil. Chop the ginger into small pieces. Mix it with the egg (broken and shell removed). Fry it with sesame oil. Eat the egg. Repeat three times a day for several days.
   - For stomach pain due to exposure to cold, add three pieces fresh ginger, 5 g white pepper powder, and 1.5 g brown sugar to hot water. Wait for 10 min. Drink the soup.
   - For stomach pain due to exposure to cold, add 9 g dried ginger, 9 g old orange peel, 12 g green onion, and 1.5 g white pepper to water. Bring to a boil for 30 min. Drink the soup.
   - For stomach pain due to exposure to cold, dry fry 60 g of Chinese prickly ash until dark in color as coal. Grind into powder. Drink it three times a day, three g each time.
   - Add 3 g Chinese prickly ash peel, 6 g dried ginger, and 12 g Xiangfu to water (500 ml). Bring to a boil for 30 to 60 min or until there is only about 200 to 300ml left. Drink the extract, once in the morning and once in the afternoon.
   - For stomach pain due to exposure to cold, fry 8 g of fennel without oil until dark in color. Drink it together with a little brown sugar.
   - For stomach pain due to exposure to cold, drink 3 g cinnamon powder with warm water.
   - For stomach pain due to exposure to cold, fry 250 g salt without oil to warm it. Fold with gauze or similar material. Apply to stomach for 10 min or until it turns cold. Replace it with a warm one. Repeat three to five times a day.

- Dry carrot seeds naturally in air. Grind them into powder. Drink the powder, 6 g each time, three times a day or whenever the stomach aches.
- Drink white radish juice after each meal, about 100 to 150 ml, with the addition of a little bit of sugar.
- Mix well 100 ml sugarcane juice and 10 ml grape wine. Drink it from time to time. Repeat for several days.
- Materials: five litchi and 50 ml liquor. Remove litchi skin, add to the liquor, add water to about 500 ml, and boil for 10 min. Drink as a tea two to three times a day. This is a one-day dose.
- Dry 100 g litchi core and 10 g old orange skin, and grind into powder. Drink as a tea two to three times a day, 10 g each time.
- Dry 100 g litchi core and 50 g costas (mu xiang), and grind into powder. Drink as a tea two to three times a day, 3 to 6 g each time.

Gastric Ulcer

1. Acupuncture is the same as for acute gastritis (see above).
2. Use folk therapy.

    - Mix 500 g honey, 62 g soda, and 48 g alumen. Bring the mixture to warm to prepare a paste. Eat one teaspoon 20 min before each meal.
    - Steam honey over water for 30 min. Eat the honey before each meal, one teaspoon each time.
    - Add 250 g each tea leaves, white sugar, and honey to 2,000 ml of water. Bring to a boil until there is about 1,000 ml left. Collect the upper clear liquid part. Store it in a clear bottle. Keep it for two weeks. Drink one to two teaspoons, once in the morning and once in the afternoon after warming it each time.

- Cut a potato into small pieces. Press to collect its juice. Drink the juice once in the morning and once in the evening, one cup each time. Continue for one month.
- Mix a half cup of tomato juice and a half cup of potato juice. Drink it twice a day for several days.
- Materials: 200 g banana and 30 g fish shell. Remove skin of banana, dry it, and grind with the fish shell into powder. Eat 3 g of powder before every meal. Repeat three times a day.

Acute Appendicitis

1. Use acupuncture on the ST36, appendix point, and ST25 points.
2. Use acupuncture on the PC3 point.
3. Use moxibustion on the Elbow-tip point.

Acute Gallstones

1. Use acupuncture on the Gallbladder point.
2. Use acupuncture on the ST36 and GB32 points.
3. Use acupuncture on the GB24 and UB18 points.
4. Use acupuncture on the Shoulder-pain two point as deep as two cun.

Roundworm in Gallbladder

1. Use acupuncture as for acute gallbladder stone.
2. Use folk therapy.
   - Mix 10 ml fresh ginger juice with 20 ml water. Drink it. Repeat after one hour. If the pain is not released, repeat every four hours until the pain is released.
   - Add several grains Chinese prickly ash peel to 60 ml vinegar. Bring to a boil for 10 min. Remove the ash peel,

and drink the vinegar. Or you can simply drink the vinegar alone after warming it a little bit. If you feel it is too sour, dilute it with water (one part to one part).
- Eat luffa seeds (black-colored ones, peeled) every day before a meal, 50 grains daily. Children should eat less.

Acute Kidney Stone

1. Use acupuncture on the Kidney-stone point (one cun above the KID3 point).
2. Use acupuncture on the hand's low-back-pain point.
3. Use acupuncture on the ST28 point.
4. Use acupuncture on the KID9 point.

Acute Intestinal Obstruction or Enteroparalysis

1. Use acupuncture on the ST36 point.
2. Use acupuncture on the ST36, ST37, and SP6 points.
3. Use acupuncture on the REN12, SP15, ST25, ST36, and PC6 points.
4. Use acupuncture on the ST35, ST37, LIV8, and PC6 points.
5. Use folk therapy.
   - For obstruction due to roundworm, mix 20 ml fresh ginger juice and 60 g honey. Drink one quart of it, and repeat the same amount every half hour.
   - Drink 150 ml sesame oil (or canola oil). Repeat the same amount once after a half hour if the condition is not corrected. If the stomach still feels bloated and painful, go to your conventional medicine doctor or Chinese medicine doctor

Incarcerated Hernia

1. Use acupuncture on the LIV1 point and then the LIV8 point.

2. Use acupuncture on the ST29 point.
3. Use folk therapy.
    - Place about 20 g of Chinese prickly ash peel in a gauze bag. Put the bag in a basin of hot water. Wash the anus with the steam. Dip the anus into the water when the water has cooled down. Do this for 20 min each time, twice a day.
    - Grind 9 g fennel and 9 g pear kernel into powder. Drink it with a little bit of cooking wine.
    - Add 9 g fennel to water. Bring to a boil for 30 min. Drink it.
    - Materials: 15 g fennel, a little salt, and two chicken eggs. Fry (without oil) the fennel and salt until dark in color. Grind them into powder. Fry the eggs (with a little oil in the frying pot) and the fennel powder. Eat the eggs every day before going to bed. Repeat every day for several days.
    - Dry eggplants (three, with bottom stems), and burn to coke. Grind the coke into powder. Drink the powder with cooking wine.
    - Bake one old luffa to dry. Grind into powder. Drink the powder three times a day, 9 g each time.
    - Material: one loquat core about 10 to 20 g. Make the core smaller, and add to water to cook as a soup. Drink the soup twice a day.

Hemorrhoids
1. Use bleeding therapy on the pile, and then do cupping on it.
2. Use acupuncture on the LU6 and UB57 points.
3. Use acupuncture on the SJ6 point.
4. Use acupuncture on the hemorrhoids point.
5. Use folk therapy.

- Eat half an orange; repeat four times a day. It can solve the constipation and stop bleeding.
- For bleeding hemorrhoids, eat a banana every morning with an empty stomach.

Heavy Cough

1. Use acupuncture on the LU6 and LU1 points.
2. Use acupuncture on the HT1 and LU5 points.
3. Use bleeding therapy on the Sifeng points (especially for child whooping cough).
4. Use folk therapy.
    - For whooping cough, prepare juice from 500 g of carrots. Add a little crystal sugar to the juice. Steam (over water) the mixture to boil. Drink it when it is warm twice a day.
    - For whooping cough, use a pear (peeled and kernel removed) and 1 g ephedra (ma huang). Add the ephedra into the hole of the pear, and steam. Remove the ephedra. Eat the pear.
    - For whooping cough, use 150 g pear (peeled and kernel removed), 30 g walnut, and 30 g rock sugar. Add to water to cook as a soup. Drink the soup every day, two to three times a day.
    - Add seven green onions (with roots), one pear, and 50 g sugar to 300 ml water. Bring to a boil until there is about 200 ml left. Drink the soup twice a day.
    - Dry luffa seeds by baking. Grind them into powder. Drink the powder, 9 g each time, three times a day.
    - Prepare juice from luffa cane. Drink the juice three times a day, 30 ml each time.
    - Bake luffa net material until dry. Grind into powder. Mix the powder with a little white sugar. Drink the mixture three times a day, 9 g each time.

- Remove the skin of two bananas and mix it with rock sugar (ground into powder). Steam over water for 20 min. Eat the banana one to two times a day for several days.
- For a cough with a little fever, use a banana root (120 g) and some salt. Grind the banana root into juice. Steam over water for 20 min, and mix with a little bit of salt. Drink the juice one to two times a day for several days.
- Materials: twenty loquats and 30 g rock sugar. Remove skin and core from the fruit, add with the sugar to 500 ml of water, and cook as a soup. Drink the soup every day for five days.
- For a hot cough, eat ten to fifteen loquats every day.
- For a hot cough, wash 40 to 60 g loquat root clean, cut into pieces, and add 100 ml water to cook as soup. Drink the soup twice a day. This is a one-day dose.
- Materials: 6 g loquat kernel, 6 g orange skin, and 6 g licorice. Wash to clean, cut into pieces, and add 1000 ml water to cook as soup until the soup is about 200 ml. Drink the soup twice a day.
- Materials: 500 g pear (peeled and kernel removed) and 500 g white lotus (cut into pieces). Prepare juices from the pear and lotus. Drink every day, three to four times a day.
- Materials: 1,000 g pear (peeled and kernel removed), 1,000 g white radish (cut into pieces), 250 g fresh ginger (make into juice), 250 g milk, and 250 g honey. Prepare juice from the pear and radish. Mix them, and add them to pot, bringing it to boiling until it looks like a paste. Add the ginger juice. Then add the milk and honey. Continue to heat to boiling. Cool down, and store the mixture in a clear bottle. Drink every day, three to four times a day.
- Materials: one pear (peeled and kernel removed, with a hole cut in it) and 6 g fritillaria (Chuan bei mu). Put the fritillaria into the pear hole. Cover the hole with its

original piece of the pear. Steam for one hour. Drink and eat it every day, three to four times a day.

- Materials: three pears (peeled and kernel removed) and 50 g honey. Grind the pear into mud form, mix with honey, and steam for one hour. Drink and eat it every day, twice a day.

- For cough and excessive phlegm, use 90 g shaddock, 15 g cooking wine, and 30 g honey. Mix them with water, and cook for about 20 to 30 min. Eat every day.

- For cough and excessive phlegm, use 90 g shaddock, 100 g pear, and 10 g rock sugar. Mix the first two with water to cook for about 20 to 30 min until they become soft. Mix them with the rock sugar. Eat every day, two to three times a day. This is used if the patient feels feverish and if the phlegm is yellow. The person should look strong, not weak, and the person does not usually feel cold in the hands or feet.

Hiccups

1. Use acupuncture on the KID1 and PC6 points.
2. Use acupuncture on the PC6, REN12, UB17, and ST36 points.
3. Put grass into the nose to cause a sneeze.
4. Press eyeballs for 2 min.
5. Press the UB2 point for 3 min.
6. Drink hot tea, and breathe deeply for 5 min.
7. Use folk therapy.

    - Mix one teaspoon sugar in two teaspoons vinegar. Swallow slowly.
    - Press Chinese chives to prepare juice. Drink the juice. Or you can just eat the Chinese chives without any cooking. Or grind the chive seeds into powder, and drink the powder.

- Press the leaves or the roots of Chinese chives into juice. Drink it every day with slow swallows. Or you can drink warm cow's milk after drinking the chive juice.
- Make juice from fresh ginger. Mix it with a little bit of honey. Drink the juice.
- Add five pumpkin stems into water. Bring to boil for 30 to sixty min. Drink the water extract.
- Mix 300 ml grape juice and fresh ginger juice. Hold a little of the mixture in the mouth. Swallow while closing the nose and ear holes with fingers. Repeat one to two times until the hiccups stop.
- Dry seven whole litchi, and grind into powder with the litchi skin. Mix with water to drink once a day.
- Burn several whole litchi (with the shell) into ash. Grind into powder. Drink the powder with water.
- Boil 10 g orange skin and 10 g fresh ginger with water. Drink the juice.
- Mix 100 ml sugarcane juice and 10 ml fresh ginger juice well. Drink it from time to time. Repeat for several days.

Aphonia

1. Use acupuncture on the KID4 point.
2. Use acupuncture on the LI18, UB13, UB12, LI11, and LI4 points (if there is no fever).
3. Use acupuncture on the REN23, DU14, LI4, LU7, and ST44 points (if there is a fever).
4. Use acupuncture on the LI18, UB13, KID3, and UB23 points (if there is a strong dry throat).
5. Use acupuncture on the REN17, PC6, REN14, and HT5 points (if it is due to a hysterical reason).

6. Use folk therapy: mix 30 g honey and 0.6 g borneol (Mei pian). Add hot water into the honey and borneol. Mix and drink it.

Nausea and Vomiting

Due to Pregnancy

1. Use acupuncture on the ST36 or SP4 points.
2. Use acupuncture on the PC6 point.
3. Use folk therapy.
   - Mix 5 ml fresh ginger juice and 10 ml honey. Drink it with the help of a drink of water afterward.
   - Hold one piece of fresh ginger under the tongue.
   - Add 60 g white sugar and 6 g fresh ginger to water (400 ml). Bring to a boil for 20 to 30 min. Drink the soup.
   - Materials: one pear (peeled and kernel removed) and 15 g liac (ding xiang). Add the liac into the hole of the pear, and steam. Remove the liac. Eat the pear.
   - Mix 100 ml fresh sugarcane juice and 20 ml fresh ginger juice well. Drink it several times a day for five to seven days.

Due to Car Sickness (or Plane Sickness or Boat Sickness)

1. Use acupuncture on the PC6 point.
2. Use acupuncture on the SJ1 and DU15 points.
3. Use the herbal tea Wuling San.

Due to Gastric Disorders

1. Use acupuncture on the REN12, ST36, PC6, SP4, and UB21 points.

2. Use acupuncture on the Stop-vomit point (0.5 cun in front of the PC7 point).
3. Use folk therapy.

    - Add 9 g fresh ginger and 9 g orange peel to water. Bring to a boil for 30 min. Drink the soup.
    - Mix fresh ginger juice and two teaspoons honey with 250 ml water. Drink all at once.
    - For toxic reaction due to ingesting chemicals, drugs, some herbs, plants, toxic seafood, and so on, use fresh ginger. Chop the ginger into a mud, or make juice from the ginger. Eat the ginger, or drink the juice.
    - For toxic reaction due to eating poisonous fish or mushrooms, use some sesame oil and 6 g alum (Bei Fan) powder. Dissolve alum into water. Drink the sesame oil to let the person vomit out the toxic residue. Then drink the alum water.
    - Materials: 40 ml potato juice, 10 drops fresh ginger juice, and one teaspoon orange juice. Mix the juices. Drink it three times a day.
    - Mix white radish juice and brown sugar, and drink it.
    - For fish poisoning, use wax gourd juice. Drink the juice in a large amount.
    - Add 10 g grape cane and 10 g fresh lotus root to water to cook for about 20 to 30 min. Drink the mixture one to two times a day.
    - Mix 30 ml grape juice and 5 ml fresh ginger juice. Drink the mixture one to two times a day.
    - Materials: 50 g fresh loquat leaves, 25 g Zhuru, 10 g cold orange skin, and 10 ml honey. Add the first three into 1000 ml water to cook as a soup until the soup is about 200 ml. Drink the soup with the addition of honey.
    - Mix 250 ml sugarcane juice and 15 ml fresh ginger juice well. Drink it all at once.

Acute Constipation

1. Use acupuncture on the SJ6 point.
2. Use acupuncture on the GB26 point.
3. Use acupuncture on the UB25, ST25, SJ6, KID6, and ST28 points.
4. Use acupuncture on the ST25, ST37, UB25, DU3, ST36, REN4, and SP6 points.
5. Use folk therapy.
   - Materials: 65 g honey and 35 ml sesame oil. Add hot water into the honey and sesame oil. Mix it well. Drink the mixture once in the morning and once in the evening. You can also simply drink the honey if there is no sesame oil available. Or you can add honey in salt water to drink every morning with an empty stomach.
   - Drink sesame oil (50 ml) in the morning or before going to bed.

Note:

1. It is better to have a Chinese medicine diagnosis to choose more precise points. The acupuncture points above are used in addition with the LI11 and LI4 points for fire-type constipation; with REN12 and LIV3 for Qi-stagnation; with UB20, UB21, and ST36 for Qi-blood deficiency; and with REN6 and moxi on REN8 points for cold-deficiency conditions.
2. If the constipation is with a high fever, such as seen in the peak time of many infectious diseases, it is better to consider Chinese herbal therapy as well. In this case, the high fever is hard to reduce without clearing the stool from the abdomen.

Acute Diarrhea

1. Use acupuncture on the HT7 and UB25 points.
2. Use acupuncture on the REN12, ST25, ST36, SP9, and ST37 points.
3. If acute diarrhea is too heavy, and the regular therapy fails to stop the diarrhea, give the herbal tea Xiao Jianzhong Tang plus Chao Baizhu, Banxia Xiexin Tang plus Chao Baishu, or Wumei Tang plus Chao Baizhu.[14]
4. Use moxibustion on the UB25, DU2, REN3, REN4, ST28, and REN9 points.
5. Use folk therapy.

    - Chop garlic into mud. Apply it into the navel, and smear it in the middle of the sole. Also, eat several pieces of garlic two to three times a day.
    - Cook an egg (remove the shell) in cooking vinegar (about 100 ml) until the egg is edible. Eat the egg.
    - Cut fresh ginger into small pieces. Add a little cooking oil in the fry pot. Fry four eggs with the ginger. Eat the fried eggs. Then drink a cup of brown sugar water.
    - Add 9 g fresh ginger and 9 g green tea leaves to water. Bring to a boil for 30 min. Drink the soup.
    - Press luffa cane and leaves to collect juice. Drink the juice three times a day.
    - For intestine inflammation, use 9 to 12 g Chinese prickly ash peel and 15 to 20 g brown sugar. Add to water (500 ml). Bring to a boil for 30 to 60 min or until there is only about 200 to 300 ml left. Drink the extract once in the morning and once in the afternoon.
    - For dysentery, use cucumber vine and leaves. Add them to water. Bring them to a boil. Drink it.

---

14. The Chao Baizhu in these formulas means the herb Baizhu is fried with another herb: Chishizhi powder.

- For dysentery, use 95 g fresh cucumber and 30 g dry cucumber vine. Add the material to water. Bring it to a boil. Drink it twice a day.
- For bacillary dysentery, use 250 g fresh grapes and 10 g brown sugar. Make the grapes into juice, and mix with the sugar. Drink the mixture all at once.

Acute Urinary Retention

1. Use acupuncture on the SP6 point.
2. Use acupuncture on the REN2, REN4, SP6, and ST28 points, plus one or two of the following points: REN3, UB23, SP9, UB28, UB32, REN6, DU20, and DU14 points.
3. Use acupuncture on the Weibao, GB28, REN6, REN4, and REN3 points, plus one or two of the following points: ST28, SP9, and SP6.
4. Use acupuncture on the REN8, ST36, REN3, UB28, and SP6 points.
5. Use acupuncture on the REN3 point (especially after birth delivery).
6. Use moxibustion on the REN8, ST36, REN3, UB28, and SP6 points. Use indirect moxibustion with a piece of fresh ginger over the points.
7. Put a warm compress on the lower abdomen and the perineum region with a warm water bag (fold with a towel) or something such as a hot-fried salt bag.
8. Massage the lower abdomen area, slightly at first and then gradually harder. Use a finger to press and massage the REN4 point.
9. Use folk therapy.
    - Grind one garlic, 6 g sanzhizi (herb), and 60 g salt into powder. Mix with water to prepare a paste. Apply the

paste into the navel. Seal it with medical tape. Keep for several hours.

- Cut fresh ginger into pieces. Apply two pieces into the navel. Fold with medical tape.
- Chop 500 g green onion into mud. Mix it with 500 g salt. Bring to a warm temperature. Fold into gauze. Apply to the lower stomach area. If it turns cold, rewarm it and apply it again. Repeat several times a day.
- For urinary cessation during pregnancy, use one cup honey and wax gourd juice. Mix the honey and the gourd juice. Drink it.

Fishbone Stuck in Throat

Use folk therapy.

- Press the LIV3 point for several min.
- Hold a vitamin C tablet (or a piece of orange skin) in the mouth for a while. Swallow saliva slowly.
- Cut garlic into thin pieces, put them into the nostrils, hold a teaspoon of white sugar in the mouth, and swallow the sugar slowly (do not drink water).
- Grind 10 g of the herb Longgu into powder. Drink it with water.
- Add the herb Weilingxian, plum, cooking vinegar, and white sugar to water, and boil until the plum becomes soft. Drink the water.
- Get a duck. Hold it with its head down. Collect its saliva. Drink the saliva (it's better to not let the patient know) with water. The fishbone can be dissolved in the duck saliva very quickly.
- Get another fishbone from the same fish, and burn it into ash. Drink the ash with warm water.

- Drink vinegar slowly. It makes the bone softer. Then drink more warm water, and then eat food.
- Blend orange skin into juice. Swallow the juice slowly.

Heavy Asthma

1. Use acupuncture on the LU10 point (toward the PC8 direction).
2. Use acupuncture on the REN17, LU7, UB13, and LU5 points.
3. Use moxibustion on the DU14, UB12, UB13, and REN17 points.
4. Use cupping on the UB13 and REN17 points.
5. Use folk therapy.
    - Add 60 g purple-skin garlic and 90 g brown sugar to 300 ml water. Bring to a boil until the mixture turns into paste. Eat the garlic paste twice a day, one teaspoon each time.
    - Fry one chicken egg with 15 g chopped ginger. Eat the egg.
    - Mix 30 g fresh ginger juice and 65 g honey. Drink the mixture three times a day with the addition of boiled water in the mixture (wait for a while for the mixture to cool down). This is a one-day dose.
    - Chop several luffa with cane, and add it to water. Bring to a boil for 30 to 60 min. Drink the water extract three times a day, one-third volume each time.
    - Prepare juice from luffa cane. Drink it each time when the asthma comes, three times a day. It can be repeated for one week.
    - Materials: one pumpkin (about 500 g), 60 ml honey, and 30 g rock sugar. Cut and open a hole in the pumpkin. Remove a little inside content from the pumpkin. Add the sugar and honey. Cover the hole again. Steam it over water for one hour. Eat the pumpkin once in the morning

and once in the evening to finish all of it. Repeat with a new pumpkin in the same way every day for several days.

- Fry (without oil) spinach seeds until yellow in color. Grind them into powder. Drink the powder twice a day, 5 g each time.
- Mix 300 ml white radish juice and 30 ml honey. Bring to a boil for 30 min. Drink it.
- Materials: 9 g apricot kernel, 20 g walnut kernel, 10 ml honey, and 10 ml fresh ginger. Remove the skin and the tip of the apricot kernel, dry frying it a little bit. Remove the skin of the walnut too. Grind the two kernels into mud. Mix with honey to prepare into a paste. Make the paste into pill form. Prepare for ten pills. Eat the pill once a day before going to bed. Drink the ginger juice to help with swallowing.
- Add 15 g apricot kernel, 15 g ephedra (Ma huan), 6 g licorice, and 250 g tofu to water to cook as a soup. Remove the ephedra. Eat the tofu and drink the soup twice a day.
- Add 50 g litchi and 10 g red tea or black tea to 300 ml of boiled water for 5 min. Drink as a tea two to three times a day.
- Mix and grind 6 g peach kernel, 6 g apricot kernel, and 6 g white pepper into powder. Prepare into a paste with egg white. Apply to the soles and the palms every night.
- Materials: 30 g shaddock skin and one *Gallus domesticus* (Wu ji).[15] Clear the feathers and inside organs from the chicken, and then insert the shaddock skin into the chicken. Fold with oil paper and then with clear soil mud. Burn the folded chicken until edible. Eat the meat once every other day.

Common Cold or Flu

15. It is a kind of chicken. Its feathers, skin, and bones are all black in color.

1. Use bleeding therapy on the DU14 point, followed by cupping.
2. Use acupuncture on the REN17 (penetrating to REN15 point) and LI3 points.
3. Use acupuncture on the common-cold point.
4. Use folk therapy.
    - Cut 15 g garlic and 15 g ginger into pieces. Add to 500 ml of water. Bring to a boil until there is about 250 ml left. Drink it before going to bed after adding a little bit of brown sugar. It is used for the cold-style common cold.
    - Add five pieces fresh ginger and 30 g brown sugar to water. Bring to a boil for 30 min. Drink the soup.
    - Add five pieces fresh ginger and one pear to water. Bring to a boil for 30 min. Drink the soup.
    - Smear fresh ginger juice on the front of the head until it feels warm. If there is a fever, smear or rub the elbow and the back of the neck.
    - Chop 60 g green onion into pieces. Add it to 300 ml water, and bring to a boil until there is about 200 ml left. Drink 100 ml when it is still warm. Drink the rest after one hour.
    - Mix 15 g green onion, 15 g fresh ginger, and 3 g salt. Grind all into mud. Fold into gauze. Rub the body (front of chest, back of chest, sole, palm, armpit, and inguinal region) with the gauze ball. After rubbing, let the person lie down to rest. It is better to have sweating after a half hour.
    - Wash cabbage roots and green onion roots, and chop into small pieces. Add them to water. Bring to a boil for 30 to 60 min to collect 500 ml of water extract. Add a little white sugar to drink it. Lie on the bed, and cover yourself with a blanket. You will feel better after sweating.

- Add 250 g cabbage inside leaves and 60 g turnip to water. Bring to a boil for 30 to 60 min. Drink the soup after the addition of a little sugar. Eat the vegetables three times a day for several days.
- Materials: 9 g apricot kernel, three pieces fresh ginger, and 100 g white radish. Remove the skin of the apricot and the radish. Add all to water, and cook as a soup. Drink the soup for several days.
- Materials: 9 g apricot kernel, 9 g mulberry leaf (sang ye), 9 g florist's chrysanthemum (Ju hua), 9 g orange stem (Ju Gen), and 9 g Arctiin. Add all to water, and cook as a soup. Drink the soup for several days.
- Make 200 g grapes into juice. Boil to make the juice stickier. Mix with a little honey. Take one tablespoon of the mixture, and mix with water to drink as a tea.
- Materials: 30 g litchi and some cooking wine. Remove the skin of the litchi, add to water, drop in some cooking wine, and boil it. Drink as a tea two to three times a day.
- Materials: 100 ml watermelon juice and 30 g reed rhizome. Add the reed rhizome to 500 ml water, and cook for 30 to 60 min. Collect the juice, and mix it with the watermelon juice. Drink the juice one to two times a day.
- Materials: 100 g watermelon skin, 30 g lalang grass rhizome, and three pieces fresh ginger. Add all to water to cook as a soup. Drink the juice twice a day.
- For the common cold in summer, use 300 g watermelon core and 300 g tomato. Make juice with gauze (not with a grinder or blender). Drink the juice from time to time every day.

Bites by Animals or Insects

Bites by Bees or Other Insects

Use folk therapy

- Chop and grind ginger into a paste. Apply to the bite.
- Chop green onion with honey into mud. Apply to the affected skin.
- Dissolve salt into water. Use the water to wash the affected skin.
- Smear soy sauce on the affected skin.
- For a bite by a scorpion (Xie Zi), mix soda with kerosene (Mei You). Prepare it into a paste. Smear the paste on the bite.
- For a bite by a mosquito, smear soda water on the affected skin.
- For a bite by a mosquito or other insect (such as a bee), smear vinegar on the skin.
- For a bite by a bee, mosquito, or snake, smear liquor on the affected skin, or mix the liquor with several drops of sesame oil, and smear it on the skin.
- For bites by bees or other insects, use about one hundred g Chinese chives and six g apricot kernel. Mix the material, and chop into a paste. Apply to the affected skin.
- For bites by bees, use the juice of an old cucumber. Smear on the skin.
- For bites by poisonous insects, grind fresh eggplant or eggplant leaves into mud. Apply to the skin. This formula can also be used for acute skin infection or skin abscess.

Bites by Snakes

Use folk therapy.

- Grind hot pepper into mud, and apply it to the bitten area. Eat fresh hot pepper at the same time.
- For skin ulcers due to a snake bite, apply fennel powder to the ulcer.

- Dilute 10 g soda with 200 ml water. Wash the bite with the soda water. Do not use this tip for broken skin.
- Grind eggplant leaves into mud. Apply it to the bite. At the same time, add eggplant leaves into water. Bring to a boil for 20 to 30 min. Drink the extract.
- Materials: luffa leaves and juice made from luffa cane and leaves. Chop 20 to 30 ml of the juice.

Bites by Dogs or Other Animals

Use folk therapy.

- For bites by dogs or rats, prepare 30 ml fresh ginger juice. Drink it. Also, grind ginger and brown sugar into a paste. Apply to the affected skin.
- Mix about 100 g Chinese chives and 6 g apricot kernel, and chop into a paste. Apply to the affected skin. Also, drink one cup Chinese chive juice.

Drunkenness

1. Use acupuncture on the REN12, PC6, and ST36 points.
2. Use folk therapy.

    - Add one to two ginger pieces and some honey (or brown sugar) to hot water. Drink the ginger water after it has cooled down.
    - Add 60 g banana skin to water to cook as a soup. Drink the soup.
    - Mix orange skin with cooking salt until it turns soft. Mix with licorice powder and sandalwood powder. Dry under sunshine. Take one tablespoon, mix with boiled water, and drink when it's cooled down.
    - Add 400 ml sugarcane juice to 200 ml boiled water. Mix well. Drink it from time to time.

- Add 30 g sugarcane skin and 30 g Gordon Euryale seed (tian shi) to water to cook as a soup. Drink it two to three times a day.

Foreign Matter in the Ear

Use folk therapy.

- Shine a light into the ear for several min. An insect in the ear may move out toward the light.
- Press Chinese chive root into juice. Insert the juice into the affected ear.
- Drop sesame oil (or other edible oil) into the ear.

Chapter 3
List of Acupuncture Points

Acupuncture point	No. of referred Fig.	Location	Acupuncture method
Bafeng (八风穴 Eight-wind point)	35	On the dorsum of the foot between the web and metatarsophalangeal joint (4 points on each foot).	Puncture subcutaneously 0.1-0.2 inch. Or puncture for bleeding.
Baihui (百会 DU20)	12	On the midline of the head, 5 cun directly above the midpoint of the anterior hairline, approximately on the midpoint of the line connecting the apexes of both ears.	Puncture subcutaneously 0.3-0.5 inch.
Baxie (八邪穴 Eight-xie point)	23	On the dorsum of the hand, at the webs between each finger, at the junction of the red & white skin.	Puncture subcutaneously 0.1-0.2 inch. Or puncture for bleeding.
Bingu (髌骨 kneecap point)	28	In a depression at the midpoint of and superior to the patella.	Puncture subcutaneously 0.3-0.5 inch.
Changqiang (长强 DU1)	13	On the midline, midway between the tip of the coccyx and the anus.	Puncture vertically 0.5-1.0 inch.
Chengjiang (承浆 REN24)	10	On the region of the face, in the depression in the center of the mentolabial groove.	Puncture obliquely upward 0.2-0.3 inch.

85

Chengshan (承山 UB57)	27	On the posterior midline of the lower leg between UB 40 and UB 60, when extending the toes straight or lifting the heel, the point is below of m. gastrocnemius in the apex of the depression.	Puncture vertically 0.8-1.2 inches.
Chimai (瘈脉 SJ18)	11	On the head, posterior to the ear in the center of the mastoid process, at the junction of the middle and lower third of the curve connecting SJ 20 and SJ 17 posterior to the helix.	Puncture subcutaneously 0.3-0.5 inch or prick with a three-edged needle to cause bleeding.
Chize (尺泽 LU5)	20	On the cubital crease of the elbow, in the depression at the radial side of the tendon of biceps brachii.	Puncture vertically 0.5-1 inch.
Chongyang (冲阳 ST42)	32	On the dome of the instep of the foot, between the tendons of long extensor muscle of the great toe and long extensor muscle of toes, where the pulsation of the dorsal artery of foot is palpable.	Avoid puncturing the artery. Puncture vertically 0.3-0.5 inch. Moxibustion is applicable.
Ciliao (次髎 UB32)	13	On the sacrum, medial and inferior to the posterosuperior iliac spine, just at the second posterior sacral foramen.	Puncture vertically 0.8-1.2 inches.
Dabai (大白穴, Big-White point)	21	On the back of hand. Between the thumb and the index finger, 1 Cun down the Linggu point.	Puncture obliquely 0.3-0.5 inch.
Dabao (大包 SP21)	14	On the mid-axillary line, in the seventh intercostal space.	Puncture obliquely 0.3-0.5 inch.
Dachangshu (大	13	1.5 cun lateral to	Puncture

肠俞 UB25)		Yaoyangguan (DU-3), at the level of the lower border of the spinous process of the fourth lumbar vertebra.	vertically 0.8-1.2 inches.
Dadun (大敦 LIV1)	32	On the lateral side of the terminal phalanx of the great toe, 0.1 cun from the corner of the nail.	Puncture subcutaneously 0.1-0.2 inch.
Daheng (大横 SP15)	15	4 cun lateral to the centre of the umbilicus, lateral to m. rectus abdominis.	Puncture vertically 0.7-1.2 inches
Daimai (带脉 GB26)	19	Directly below Zhangmen LIV-13 (anterior and inferior to the free end of the eleventh rib), level with the umbilicus.	Puncture vertically 0.5-0.8 inch.
Daling (大陵 PC7)	20	In the middle of the transverse crease of the wrist, between the tendons of m. palmaris longus and m. flexor carpi radialis.	Puncture vertically 0.3-0.5 inch.
Dannang (胆囊穴 Gall bladder point)	28	1-2 cun below GB 34 (palpate for most tender point).	Puncture vertically 0.7-1.2 inches
Danshu (胆俞 UB19)	13	1.5 cun lateral to the lower border of the spinous process of the tenth thoracic vertebra (T10).	Puncture obliquely 0.5-0.8 inch.
Dazhu (大杼 UB11)	13	1.5 cun lateral to the lower border of the spinous process of the first thoracic vertebra (T1).	Puncture obliquely 0.5-0.7 inch.
Dazhong (大钟 KID4)		Posterior and inferior to the medial malleolus, in the depression anterior to the medial side of the attachment of Achilles' tendon.	Puncture vertically 0.3-0.5 inch.

Dazhui (大椎 DU14)	13	On the midline at the base of the neck, in the depression below the spinous process of the seventh cervical vertebra.	Puncture obliquely upward 0.5-1.0 inch.
Dichang (地仓 ST4)	10	Lateral to the corner of the mouth, directly below the pupil.	Puncture subcutaneously 1.0-1.5 inches with the tip of the needle directed towards Jiache (ST 6).
Dubi (犊鼻 ST35)	28	When the knee is flexed, the point is at the lower border of the patella, in the depression lateral to the patellar ligament.	Puncture vertically 0.7-1.0 inch.
Duyin (独阴 Single-Yin point)	34	On the sole side of foot, In the middle of the second line of toe joints.	Puncture subcutaneously 0.1-0.2 inch.
Erbai (二白穴 Two-white point)	20	4 cun above the wrist crease, proximal to PC 7 on both sides of the flexor carpi radialis tendon.	Puncture vertically 0.2-0.3 inch.
Erjian (二间 LI2)	21	On the radial border of the index finger, in a depression just distal to the metacarpo-phalangeal joint.	Puncture vertically 0.2-0.3 inch.
Fengchi (风池 GB20)	12	Below the occiput, approximately midway between Fengfu DU-16 and Wangu GB-12, in the hollow between the origins of the sternomastoid and trapezius muscles.	Puncture subcutaneously 0.3-0.5 inch.
Fengshi (风市 GB31)	26	On the lateral aspect of the thigh, directly below the greater trochanter, 7 cun	Puncture vertically 0.7-1.2 inches.

			superior to the popliteal crease.	
Feiping (肺平穴 Lung-ease point)		20	On the palm side of front arm. Upper one third between elbow and wrist line.	Puncture vertically 0.7-1.2 inches.
Feishu (肺俞 UB13)		13	1.5 cun lateral to the lower border of the spinous process of the third thoracic vertebra (T3).	Puncture obliquely 0.5-0.7 inch.
Fengfu (风府 DU16)		12	On the midline at the nape of the neck, in the depression immediately below the external occipital protuberance.	Puncture vertically 0.5-0.8 inch. Deep puncture is not advisable. Medullary bulb is in the deep layer, special attention should be paid in acupuncture.
Fenglong (丰隆 ST40)		28	8 cun superior to the tip of the external malleolus, lateral to Tiaokou (ST-38) about two finger-breadth lateral to the anterior border of the tibia.	Puncture vertically 0.5-1.0 inch.
Fengmen (风门 UB12)		12	1.5 cun lateral to the lower border of the spinous process of the second thoracic vertebra (T2).	Puncture obliquely 0.5-0.7 inch.
Fuling point (妇灵穴)		34	On the sole side of foot, the two sides of the root of the second toe (2 points on each foot)	Puncture subcutaneously 0.1-0.2 inch.
Fuliu (复溜 KID7)		20	2 cun directly above Taixi (KI-3), on the anterior border of Achilles' tendon.	Puncture vertically 0.5-0.7 inch.

Futu (扶突 LI18)	11	On the lateral side of the neck, level with the tip of the laryngeal prominence, between the sternal and clavicular heads of the sternocleidomastoid muscle.	Puncture vertically 0.3-0.5 inch.
Hand Yaotong point (手腰痛穴, Back-pain ponit on hand)	21	On the dorsum of the hand, midway between the transverse wrist crease and the metacarpalphalangeal joint, between both the 2nd and 3rd and the 4th and 5th metacarpals (2 points on each hand).	Puncture vertically 0.5-0.7 inch.
Head Yaotong (头腰痛穴, Back-pain point on head)	10	On the middle of the front head	Puncture subcutaneously 0.3-0.5 inch.
Hegu (合谷 LI4)	21	On the dorsum of the hand, between the first and second metacarpal bones, at the midpoint of the second metacarpal bone and close to its radial border.	Puncture vertically 0.5-0.8 inch. Acupuncture on this point is contraindicated in pregnant women.
Herpes point (带状疱疹点)	21	On the back of 5th finger. Middle of the last joint on the finger.	Puncture vertically 0.1-0.2 inch.
Heyang (合阳 UB55)	27	On the lower leg, 2 cun inferior to Weizhong BL-40, on the line connecting Weizhong BL-40 and Chengshan BL-57, in the depression between the two heads of the gastrocnemius muscle.	Puncture vertically 0.7-1.0 inch.

Houding (后顶 DU19)	12	5.5 cun directly above the midpoint of the posterior hairline, 1.5 cun directly above Qiangjian (DU-18).	Puncture subcutaneously 0.3-0.5 inch.
Houxi (后溪 SI3)	21	On the ulnar border of the hand, in the substantial depression proximal to the head of the fifth metacarpal bone.	Puncture vertically 0.5-0.7 inch.
Huantiao (环跳 GB30)	24	On the postero-lateral aspect of the hip joint, one third of the distance between the prominence of the greater trochanter and the sacro-coccygeal hiatus (Yaoshu DU-2).	Puncture vertically 1.5-2.5 inches.
Huanzhongshang (环中上穴)	24	Bend the thigh, 2 Cun over the middle point between the tailbone and the trochiter.	Puncture vertically 1.5-2.5 inches.
Huiyang (会阳 UB35)	13	0.5 cun lateral to the Governing vessel, level with the tip of the coccyx.	Puncture vertically 0.5-1.0 inch.
Huiyi (会阴 REN1)	25	At the perineum, midway between the anus and the scrotum in men, and the anus and the posterior labial commissure in women.	Puncture vertically 0.5-1.0 inch.
Jiache (颊车 ST6)	11	Approximately 1 fingerbreadth anterior and superior to the angle of the jaw at the prominence of the masseter muscle.	Puncture vertically 0.3-0.5 inch, or subcutaneously with the tip of the needle directed towards Dicang (ST 4).

Jianbei (肩背穴 shoulder-back point)	13	4 to 5 cm beside tailbone.	Puncture vertically 1.5-2.5 inches.
Jiaji (夹脊穴)	36	A group of 34 points, .5 cun lateral to the lower border of the spinous processes of T1-L5.	Puncture vertically 0.3-0.5 inch.
Jianjing (肩井 GB21)	12	Midway between Dazhui DU-14 and the tip of the acromion, at the crest of the trapezius muscle.	Puncture vertically 0.3-0.5 inch.
Jianliao (肩髎 SJ14)	16	At the origin of the deltoid muscle, in the depression which lies posterior and inferior to the lateral extremity of the acromion.	Puncture vertically 0.7-1.0 inch.
Jianqi point (肩奇穴)	14	2 Cun from the shoulder tip, on the rear edge of collarbone.	Puncture vertically 0.3-0.5 inch. Needle towards shoulder.
Jiangtong point (肩痛穴)		Upper 1/3 spot, between the caput fibulae and the external malleolus	Puncture vertically 1.0-2.0 inch.
Jiangtong 1 point (肩痛1穴 Shoulder pain point 1)	29	0.5 Cun below the Yinlingquan point, penetrating towards Zusanli point	Puncture vertically 1.0-2.0 inch.
Jianyu (臂髃 LI15)	16	In the depression which lies anterior and inferior to the acromion, at the origin of the deltoid muscle. (Note: Jianliao SJ-14 is located in the depression which lies posterior and inferior to the acromion).	Puncture vertically or obliquely 0.8-1.5 inches.

Jianzhen (肩贞 SI9)	12	Posterior and inferior to the shoulder joint. When the arm is adducted, the point is 1 cun above the posterior end of the axillary fold.	Puncture vertically 0.5-1.0 inch.
Jianzhong (肩中)	16	On the middle of shoulder deltoid.	Puncture vertically 1.5-2.5 inches.
Jiexi (解溪 ST41)	32	On the ankle, level with the prominence of the lateral malleolus, in a depression between the tendons of extensor hallucis longus and extensor digitorum longus.	Puncture vertically 0.5-0.7 inch.
Jinqu (经渠 LU8)	20	1 cun above the transverse crease of the wrist in the depression on the lateral side of the radial artery.	Puncture vertically 0.1-0.3 inch. Avoid puncturing the radial artery.
Jingmen (京门 GB25)	15	Below the lateral aspect of the ribcage, anterior and inferior to the free end of the 12th rib.	Puncture vertically 0.3-0.5 inch.
Jingming (睛明 UB1)	10	0.1 cun medial and superior to the inner canthus of the eye, near the medial border of the orbit.	Ask the patient to close his eyes when pushing gently the eyeball to the lateral side. Puncture slowly vertically 0.3-0.7 inch along the orbital wall. It is not advisable to twist of lift and thrust the needle vigorously. To avoid bleeding,

				press the puncturing site for a few seconds after withdrawal of the needle. Moxibustion is forbidden.
Jinsuo (筋缩 DU8)	13		Below the spinous process of the ninth thoracic vertebra.	Puncture vertically 0.5-1.0 inch.
Jiquan (极泉 HT1)	19		When the upper arm is abducted, the point is in the centre of the axilla, on the medial side of the axillary artery.	Avoid puncturing the axillary artery. Puncture vertically 0.5-1.0 inch.
Jiuwei (鸠尾 REN15)	14		On the anterior midline, 1 cun below the xiphosternal synchondrosis. Locate the point in supine position with the arms uplifted.	Puncture obliquely downward 0.4-0.6 inch.
Jizhudian (脊椎点)	21		Between the Qiangu and Houxi, on the joint line.	Puncture vertically 0.3-0.8 inch.
Juque (巨阙 REN14)	15		On the midline of the abdomen, 6 cun above the umbilicus and 2 cun below the sternocostal angle.	Puncture vertically 0.3-0.8 inch.
Kidney stone point (肾结石点)	29		1 Cun above the Taixi point.	Puncture vertically 0.5-1 inch.
Kongzui (孔最 LU6)	20		On the flexor aspect of the forearm, 7 cun proximal to Taiyuan LU-9, on the line connecting Taiyuan LU-9 with Chize LU-5.	Puncture vertically 0.5-1 inch.

Kuangu (髋骨穴)	28,30	1.5 Cun away from the Liangqiu points, two points on each knee。	Puncture vertically 0.5-1 inch.
Kunlun (昆仑 UB60)	31	Behind the ankle joint, in the depression between the prominence of the lateral malleolus and the Achilles tendon.	Puncture vertically 0.5-1.0 inch.
Ganmao point (感冒穴)	21	Between the metacarpophalangeal joints of the middle finger and the 4th finger, between the white and red skin edge.	Puncture vertically 3-4 cm towards the wrist direction.
Ganshu (肝俞 UB18)	13	1.5 cun lateral to the lower border of the spinous process of the ninth thoracic vertebra (T9).	Puncture obliquely 0.5-0.7 inch.
Gaohuan (膏肓 UB43)	12	3 cun lateral to the Governor Vessel, at the level of the lower border of the spinous process of the fourth thoracic vertebra, on the spinal border of the scapula.	Puncture vertically 0.3-0.5 inch.
Geshu (膈俞 UB17)	13	1.5 cun lateral to the lower border of the spinous process of the seventh thoracic vertebra (T7).	Puncture obliquely 0.5-0.7 inch.
Gongson (公孙 SP4)	33	On the medial side of the foot, in the depression distal and inferior to the base of the first metatarsal bone.	Puncture vertically 0.5-0.8 inch.

Guanyuan (关元 REN4)	15	On the midline of the lower abdomen, 3 cun inferior to the umbilicus and 2 cun superior to the pubic symphysis.	Puncture vertically 0.8-1.2 inches. Great care should be taken to puncture the points from Qugu (REN-02) to Shangwan (REN-13) of this meridian in pregnant women. Moxibustion is applicable.
Guanxin (冠心穴)	32	On foot back, 2.5 Cun down from Jiexi point.	Puncture vertically 0.5-0.8 inch.
Guanchong (关冲 SJ1)	21	On the lateral side of the ring finger, about 0.1 cun from the corner of the nail.	Puncture superficially 0.1 inch, or prick with a three-edged needle to cause bleeding.
Guilai (归来 ST29)	15	4 cun below the umbilicus, 2 cun lateral to Zhongji (REN-3).	Puncture vertically 0.7-1.2 inches.
Lanwei point (兰尾穴)	28	2 cun below Zusanli.	Puncture vertically 1-2 inches.
Laogong (劳宫 PC8)	20	Between the second and third metacarpal bones, proximal to the metacarpo-phalangeal joint, in a depression at the radial side of the third metacarpal bone.	Puncture vertically 0.3-0.5 inch.

Lidui (历兑 ST45)	32	On the lateral side of the 2nd toe, 0.1 cun posterior to the corner of the nail.	Puncture subcutaneously 0.1 inch.
Liangmen (梁门 ST21)	15	4 cun above the umbilicus, 2 cun lateral to Zhongwan (REN-12).	Puncture vertically 0.8-1.0 inch.
Liangqiu (梁丘 ST34)	30	When the knee is flexed, the point is 2 cun above the laterosuperior border of the patella.	Puncture vertically 0.5-1.0 inch.
Lianquan (廉泉 REN23)	11	Above the Adam's apple, in the depression of the upper border of the hyoid bone.	Puncture obliquely 0.5-1.0 inch toward the tongue root.
Lieque (列缺 LU7)	20	On the radial aspect of the forearm, approximately 1.5 cun proximal to Yangxi L.I.-5, in the cleft between the tendons of brachioradialis and abductor pollicis longus.	Puncture 0.3-0.5 inch obliquely upward.
Ligou (蠡沟 LIV5)	29	5 cun above the tip of the medial malleolus, on the midline of the medial surface of the tibia.	Puncture subcutaneously 0.3-0.5 inch.
Linggu (灵骨穴)	21	On the back of hand, between the first and the second metacarpale.	Puncture vertically 0.5-1.0 inch.
Menjin (门金)	32	On the back of foot, ankle side of between the 2nd and 3th metatarsal bones.	Puncture vertically 0.3-0.5 inch.
Mingmen (命门 DU4)	13	On the midline of the lower back, in the depression below the spinous process of the second lumbar vertebra.	Puncture vertically 0.5-1.0 inch.

Name	No.	Location	Needling
Neiguan (内关 PC6)	20	On the flexor aspect of the forearm, 2 cun proximal to Daling P-7, between the tendons of palmaris longus and flexor carpi radialis.	Puncture vertically 0.5-0.8 inch.
Neiting (内庭 ST44)	32	Proximal to the web margin between the 2nd and 3rd toes, in the depression distal and lateral to the 2nd metatarsodigital joint.	Puncture vertically 0.3-0.5 inch.
Niushang (扭伤穴)	27	Middle point between the Chengshan point and the bottom of the heel.	Puncture vertically 1-2 inches.
Qihai (气海 REN6)	15	On the anterior midline, 1.5 cun below the umbilicus.	Puncture vertically 0.8-1.2 inches. Great care should be taken to puncture the points from Qugu (REN-02) to Shangwan (REN-13) of this meridian in pregnant women.
Qiuxu (丘墟 GB40)	31	At the ankle joint, in the depression anterior and inferior to the lateral malleolus.	Puncture vertically 0.5-0.8 inch.
Quanliao (颧髎 SI18)	11	Directly below the outer canthus, in the depression at the lower border of the zygomatic bone.	Puncture vertically 0.5-0.8 inch.
Quchi (曲池 LI11)	16,18	At the elbow, midway between Chize LU-5 and the lateral epicondyle of the humerus, at the lateral end of	Puncture vertically 1.0-1.5 inches.

			the transverse cubital crease.	
Qugu (曲骨 REN2)	15		On the midline of the lower abdomen, at the superior border of the pubic symphysis, 5 cun below the umbilicus.	Puncture vertically 0.5-1.0 inch. Great care should be taken to puncture the points from Qugu (REN-02) to Shangwan (REN-13) of this meridian in pregnant women.
Quze (曲泽 PC3)	20		On the transverse cubital crease, at the ulnar side of the tendon of m. biceps brachii.	Puncture vertically 0.5-0.7 inch, or prick with a three-edged needle to cause bleeding.
Pangguangshu (膀胱俞 UB28)	13		1.5 cun lateral to the midline, at the level of the second posterior sacral foramen.	Puncture vertically 0.8-1.2 inches.
Pishu (脾俞 UB20)	13		1.5 cun lateral to the lower border of the spinous process of the eleventh thoracic vertebra (T11).	Puncture obliquely 0.5-0.7 inch.
Piantan (偏瘫穴 paralysis point)	11		3 cm over the ear tip	Puncture obliquely 0.5-0.7 inch.
Rangu (然谷 KID2)	33		Anterior and inferior to the medial malleolus, in the depression on the lower border of the tuberosity of the navicular bone.	Puncture vertically 0.3-0.5 inch.
Renzhong (水沟 DU26)	10		At the junction of the upper third and middle third of the philtrum.	Puncture obliquely upward 0.3-0.5 inch.

Riyue (日月 GB24)	14	On the anterior chest wall, in the seventh intercostal space, directly below the nipple, 4 cun lateral to the midline.	Puncture obliquely 0.3-0.5 inch.
Sanjian (三间 LI3)	21	On the radial side of the index finger, in the substantial depression proximal to the head of the second metacarpal bone.	Puncture vertically 0.5-0.8 inch.
Sanyinjiao (三阴交 SP6)	29	3 cun directly above the tip of the medial malleolus, posterior to the medial border of the tibia.	Puncture vertically 0.5-1.0 inch
Sanyinjiao Hou point (三阴交后穴)	29	the same level as Sanyinjiao, on the front edge of Achilles tendon (the pressing pain point)	Puncture vertically 0.5-1.0 inch
Sanmao (三毛穴 three-hair point)	32	On the back of the end stem of the big toe	Puncture vertically 0.1-0.2 inch
Shanzhong (膻中穴 REN17)	14	On the anterior midline, at the level with the fourth intercostal space, midway between the nipples.	Puncture subcutaneously 0.3-0.5 inch.
Shandian (闪电穴 thunder-flash point)	13	6 Cun beside the tip of tailbone.	Puncture vertically 3-4 inches.
Shangdu (上都)	23	Between the metacarpophalangeal joints of the second finger and the 3th finger, between the white and red skin edge.	Puncture subcutaneously 0.3-0.5 inch.
Shangjuxu (上巨虚 ST37)	28	On the lower leg, 3 cun inferior to Zusanli ST-36, one finger-breadth lateral to the anterior crest of the tibia.	Puncture vertically 0.5-1.2 inches.

Point		Location	Needling
Shangyang (商阳 LI1)	23	On the dorsal aspect of the index finger, at the junction of lines drawn along the radial border of the nail and the base of the nail, approximately 0.1 cun from the corner of the nail.	Puncture 0.1 inch, or prick the point to cause bleeding.
Shangxing (上星 DU23)	10	1 cun directly above the midpoint of the anterior hairline.	Puncture subcutaneously 0.3-0.5 inch or prick to cause bleeding.
Shaofu (少府 HT8)	22	On the palm, in the depression between the 4th and 5th metacarpal bones, where the tip of the little finger rests when a fist is made.	Puncture vertically 0.3-0.5 inch.
Shaoshang (少商 LU11)	23	On the extensor aspect of the thumb, at the junction of lines drawn along the radial border of the nail and the base of the nail, approximately 0.1 cun from the corner of the nail.	Puncture 0.1 inch, or prick the point to cause bleeding.
Shaohai (少海 HT3)	21	Midway between Quze P-3 and the medial epicondyle of the humerus, at the medial end of the transverse cubital crease when the elbow is fully flexed.	Puncture vertically 0.5-1.0 inch.
Shenmen (神门 HT7)	22	At the ulnar end of the transverse crease of the wrist, in the depression on the radial side of the tendon of m. flexor carpi ulnaris.	Puncture vertically 0.3-0.5 inch.
Shenmai (申脉 UB62)	31	On the lateral side of the foot, approximately 0.5 cun inferior to the inferior border of the	Puncture vertically 0.3-0.5 inch.

		lateral malleolus, in a depression posterior to the peroneal tendons.	
Shenque (神阙 REN8)	15	In the centre of the umbilicus.	Puncture is prohibited. Great care should be taken to puncture the points from Qugu (REN-02) to Shangwan (REN-13) of this meridian in pregnant women.
Shenshu (肾俞 UB23)	13	1.5 cun lateral to Mingmen (DU-4), at the level of the lower border of the spinous process of the second lumbar vertebra.	Puncture vertically 1-1.2 inches.
Shenting (神庭 DU24)	10	0.5 cun directly above the midpoint of the anterior hairline.	Puncture subcutaneously 0.3-0.5 inch, or prick to cause bleeding.
Shouqianjin (手千金)	17	Outside of ulna, 7.5 Cun from the transverse striation of wrist.	Puncture vertically 0.3-1 inch.
Shousanli (手三里 LI10)	16	On the line joining Yangxi (LI-5) and Quchi (LI-11), 2 cun below the cubital crease.	Puncture vertically 0.8-1.2 inches.
Shouwujin (手五金)	17	Outside of ulna, 6.5 Cun from the transverse striation of wrist.	Puncture vertically 0.3-1 inch.
Shouwuli (手五里 LI13)	16	On the lateral side of the upper arm, 3 cun proximal to Quchi L.I.-11, on the line connecting Quchi L.I.-11 with Jianyu L.I.-	Puncture vertically 0.5-1.0 inch. Avoid injuring the artery.

			15.
Shuaigu (率谷 GB8)	11	In the temporal region, in the slight depression 1 cun directly above the apex of the ear.	Puncture subcutaneously 0.3-0.5 inch.
Shuidao (水道 ST28)	15	3 cun below the umbilicus, 2 cun lateral to Guanyuan (REN-4).	Puncture vertically 0.7-1.2 inches.
Shuifen (水分 REN9)	15	On the anterior midline, 1 cun above the umbilicus.	Puncture vertically 0.5-1.0 inch. Great care should be taken to puncture the points from Qugu (REN-02) to Shangwan (REN-13) of this meridian in pregnant women.
Sibai (四白 ST2)	10	Directly below the pupil, in the depression at the infraorbital foramen.	Puncture vertically 0.2-0.3 inch. It is not advisable to puncture deeply.
Sifeng (四缝)	22	Midpoint of the crease of each proximal interphalangeal joint.	Puncture subcutaneously 0.1-0.2 inch.
Shixuan (十宣穴)	22	Tips of fingers.	Puncture subcutaneously 0.1-0.2 inch.
Sizhi (四肢穴)	29	1.5 Cun under the Yinlingquan	Puncture vertically 0.5-1 inch.
Stomach pain (胃痛穴 stomach-	10	1 Cun under the mouth edge.	Puncture vertically or

pain point)			obliquely 0.2-3 inch.
Suliao (素髎 DU25)	10	On the midline at the tip of the nose.	Puncture perpendicularly 0.2-0.3 inch, or prick to cause bleeding.
Taibai (太白 SP3)	33	On the medial side of the foot in the depression proximal and inferior to the head of the first metatarsal bone.	Puncture vertically 0.3-0.5 inch.
Taichong (太冲 LIV3)	32	On the dorsum of the foot, in the hollow distal to the junction of the first and second metatarsal bones.	Puncture vertically 0.3-0.5 inch.
Taixi (太溪 KID3)	33	In the depression between the tip of the medial malleolus and Achilles' tendon.	Puncture vertically 0.3-0.5 inch.
Taiyuan (太渊 LU9)	20	At the wrist joint, in the depression between the radial artery and the tendon of abductor pollicis longus, level with Shenmen HE-7 (the proximal border of the pisiform bone).	Puncture vertically 0.2-0.3 inch. Avoid puncturing the radial artery.
Tianfu (天府 LU3)	14	On the medial aspect of the upper arm, 3 cun below the end of axillary fold, on the radial side of m. biceps brachii.	Puncture vertically 0.5-1 inch.
Tianjin (天井 SJ10)	18	With the elbow flexed, this point is located in the depression 1 cun proximal to the olecranon.	Puncture vertically 0.3-0.5 inch.

Point		Location	Puncture
Tianzong (天宗 SI11)	12	On the scapula, in a tender depression one third of the distance from the midpoint of the inferior border of the scapular spine to the inferior angle of the scapula.	Puncture vertically or obliquely 0.5-1.0 inch.
Tianshu (天枢 ST25)	15	On the abdomen, 2 cun lateral to the umbilicus.	Puncture vertically 0.7-1.2 inches.
Tianzhu (天柱 UB10)	12	On the lateral aspect of the trapezius muscle, 1.3 cun lateral to Yamen DU-15.	Puncture vertically 0.5-0.8 inch.
Tiantu (天突 REN22)	14	In the centre of the suprasternal fossa.	First puncture vertically 0.2 inch and then insert the needle tip downward along the posterior aspect of the sternum 0.5-1.0 inch.
Tingong (听宫 SI19)	11	With the mouth open, this point is located in the depression between the middle of the tragus and the condyloid process of the mandible.	Puncture vertically 0.5-1.0 inch when the mouth is open.
Tiaokou (条口 ST38)	28	8 cun below Dubi (ST-35), and one finger breadth (middle finger) from the anterior border of the tibia.	Puncture vertically 0.5-1.0 inch.
Tongli (通里 HT5)	22	When the palm faces upward, the point is on the radial side of the tendon of m. flexor carpi ulnaris, 1 cun above the transverse crease of the wrist.	Puncture vertically 0.3-0.5 inch.

Tuntong (臀痛点)	12	Middle of the rear line of armpit	Puncture vertically 0.5-1 inch.
Tongziliao (童子髎 GB1)	10	In the hollow on the lateral side of the orbital margin, approximately 0.5 cun lateral to the outer canthus.	Puncture subcutaneously 0.3-0.5 inch.
Under-tongue (舌下穴)	37	On the veins on either side of the frenulum of the tongue - Jinjin is on the Left side and Yuye is on the Right side.	Puncture to cause bleeding
Waiguan (外关 SJ5)	17	2 cun proximal to Yangchi SJ-4, in the depression between the radius and the ulna, on the radial side of the extensor digitorum communis tendons.	Puncture vertically 0.5-1.0 inch.
Weibao (维胞穴)	15	3 Cun under the navel, then 6 Cun aside. Just in front and little bit down of anterior superior spine.	Puncture vertically 1-2 inches.
Weidao (维道 GB28)	15	Anterior and inferior to the anterior superior iliac spine, 0.5 cun anterior and inferior to Wushu (GB-27).	Puncture vertically 0.5-1.0 inch.
Weishu (胃俞 UB21)	13	1.5 cun lateral to the lower border of the spinous process of the twelfth thoracic vertebra (T12).	Puncture obliquely 0.5-0.8 inch.
Stomach pain point	10	1 Cun under the edge of mouth.	Puncture obliquely 0.5-0.8 inch.
Weizhong (委中 UB40)	27	At the back of the knee, on the popliteal crease, in a depression midway between the tendons of biceps femoris and semitendinosus.	Puncture vertically 0.5-1.0 inch, or prick the popliteal vein with three-edged

			needle to cause bleeding.
Xiabai (侠白 LU4)	14	On the medial aspect of the upper arm, 4 cun below the anterior end of the axillary fold, or 5 cun above the cubital crease, on the radial side of m. biceps brachii.	Puncture vertically 0.5-1 inch.
Xiaguan (下关 ST7)	11	On the face, anterior to the ear, in the depression between the zygomatic arch and the mandibular notch. This point is located with the mouth closed.	Puncture vertically 0.3-0.5 inch.
Xialian (下廉 LI8)	18	On the line joining Yangxi (LI-5) and Quchi (LI-11), 4 cun below the cubital crease.	Puncture vertically 0.5-1.0 inch.
Xiaohai (小海 SI8)	20	In the depression between the tip of the olecranon process of the ulna and the tip of the medial epicondyle of the humerus.	Puncture vertically 0.3-0.5 inch.
Xiangu (陷谷 ST43)	32	In the depression distal to the junction of the 2nd and 3rd metatarsal bones.	Puncture vertically 0.3-0.5 inch.
Xiaogukong (小骨空)	21	On the back of hand, on the middle of the first finger joint of the 5th finger.	Puncture obliquely 0.1-0.2 inch.

Xiawan (下脘 REN10)	15	On the anterior midline, 2 cun above the umbilicus.	Puncture vertically 0.5-1.2 inches. Great care should be taken to puncture the points from Qugu (REN-02) to Shangwan (REN-13) of this meridian in pregnant women.
Xiguan point (膝关穴 Knee-gate point)	29	1 to 1.5 Cun the back of Yinlingquan point	Puncture vertically 1-2 inches.
Xinshu (心俞 UB15)	13	1.5 cun lateral to the lower border of the spinous process of the fifth thoracic vertebra (T5).	Puncture obliquely 0.5-0.7 inch.
Xingjian (行间 LIV2)		On the dorsum of the foot between the first and second toe, proximal to the margin of the web at the junction of the red and white skin.	Puncture obliquely 0.3-0.5 inch.
Xingnao point (醒脑穴 brain-wake point)	11	On the hollow between cleidomastoid and cucullaris upper part.	Puncture obliquely 0.3-0.5 inch.
Xiongtong (胸痛穴 chest-pain point)	18	On the back of front arm. One thid of the line between the wrist and elbow, to the wrist side.	Puncture vertically 1-2 inches.
Xiyangguan (膝阳关 GB33)	28	On the lateral side of the knee, in the depression above the lateral epicondyle of the femur, between the femur and tendon of biceps femoris.	Puncture vertically 0.5-1.0 inch.

Xuanzhong (悬钟 GB39)	31	Above the ankle joint, 3 cun superior to the prominence of the lateral malleolus, between the posterior border of the fibula and the tendons of peroneus longus and brevis.	Puncture vertically 0.3-0.5 inch.
Xuehai (血海 SP10)	30	When the knee is flexed, the point is 2 cun above the medio-superior border of the patella, on the bulge of the medial portion of m. quadriceps femoris.	Puncture vertically 0.5-1.2 inches.
Yangchi (阳池 SJ4)	21	On the dorsum of the wrist, at the level of the wrist joint, in the depression between the tendons of extensor digitorum communis and extensor digiti minimi.	Puncture vertically 0.3-0.5 inch.
Yangfu (阳辅 GB38)	26	On the lateral aspect of the lower leg, 4 cun superior to the prominence of the lateral malleolus, at the anterior border of the fibula.	Puncture vertically 0.5-0.7 inch.
Yanglao (养老 SI6)	21	Dorsal to the head of the ulna. When tile palm face the chest, the point is in the bony cleft on radial side of the styloid process of the ulna.	Puncture vertically 0.3-0.5 inch.
Yangxi (阳溪 LI5)	21	On the radial side of the wrist. When the thumb is tilted upward, it is in the depression between the tendons m. extensor pollicis longus and brevis.	Puncture vertically 0.3-0.5 inch.

Name		Location	Puncture
Yamen (哑门 DU15)	12	0.5 cun directly above the midpoint of the posterior hairline, in the depression below the spinous process of the first cervical vertebra.	Puncture vertically 0.5-0.8 inch. Neither upward obliquely nor deep puncture is advisable. It is near the medullary bulb in the deep layer, and the depth and angle of the puncture should be paid strict attention to.
Yaoshu (腰俞 DU2)	13	In the hiatus of the sacrum.	Puncture obliquely upward 0.5-1.0 inch.
Yaoqi (腰奇穴 lower-back mystery point)	13	2 Cun above the tailtip.	Puncture vertically 1-1.5 inch.
Yaoyangguan (腰阳关 DU3)	13	On the midline of the lower back, in the depression below the spinous process of the fourth lumbar vertebra.	Puncture vertically 0.5-1.0 inch.
Yatong point (牙痛穴 Toothache point)	11	Before ear drop, on the rear edge of angle of the jaw.	Puncture vertically 0.5-1.0 inch.
Yinbai (隐白 SP1)	33	On the medial side of the great toe, 0.1 cun posterior to the corner of the nail.	Puncture subcutaneously 0.1 inch.
Yinmen (殷门 UB37)	27	6 cun below Chengfu (BL-36) on the line joining Chengfu (BL-36) and Weizhong (BL-40).	Puncture vertically 1.0-2.0 inches.

Name		Location	Puncture
Yinlingquan (阴陵泉 SP9)	29	On the lower border of the medial condyle of the tibia, in the depression posterior and inferior to the medial condyle of the tibia.	Puncture vertically 0.5-1.0 inch.
Yintang (印堂)	10	Midway between the medial ends of the eyebrows	Puncture subcutaneously 0.1 inch.
Yinxiang (迎香 LI20)	10	In the naso-labial groove, at the level of the midpoint of the lateral border of the ala nasi.	Puncture obliquely or subcutaneously 0.3-0.5 inch.
Yongquan (涌泉 KID1)	34	On the sole of the foot, between the second and third metatarsal bones, approximately one third of the distance between the base of the second toe and the heel, in a depression formed when the foot is plantar flexed.	Puncture vertically 0.3-0.5 inch.
Yuji (鱼际 LU10)	20	On the thenar eminence of the hand, in a depression between the midpoint of the shaft of the first metacarpal bone and the thenar muscles.	Puncture vertically 0.5-0.8 inch.
Yunmen (云门 LU2)	14	On the antero-lateral aspect of the chest, below the lateral extremity of the clavicle, 6 cun lateral to the midline, in the center of the hollow of the delto-pectoral triangle.	Puncture obliquely 0.5-0.8 inch towards the lateral aspect of the chest. To avoid injuring the lung, never puncture deeply towards the medial aspect.

Name		Description	Puncture
Zanzhu (攒竹 UB2)	10	Superior to the inner canthus, in a depression on the eyebrow, close to its medial end.	Puncture subcutaneously 0.3-0.5 inch, or prick with three-edged needle to cause bleeding.
Zhaohai (照海 KID6)	33	In the depression below the tip of the medial malleolus.	Puncture vertically 0.3-0.5 inch.
Zhibian (秩边 UB54)	13	On the buttock, in the depression 3 cun lateral to the sacro-coccygeal hiatus.	Puncture vertically 1.5-2.0 inches.
Zhicuang point (痔疮穴 haemorrhoids point)	17	On the back of front arm, one third between the wrist and the elbow line, towards elbow side.	Puncture vertically 1-1.5 inches.
Zhigou (支沟 SJ6)	17	3 cun proximal to Yangchi SJ-4, in the depression between the radius and the ulna, on the radial side of the extensor digitorum communis muscle.	Puncture vertically 0.8-1.2 inches.
Zhiou point (止呕穴 stop-vomit point)	20	0.5 Cun in front of Daling point (0.5 Cun to the wrist line)	Puncture vertically 0.3-0.5 inch.
Zhiyin (至阴 UB67)	31	On the lateral side of the small toe, about 0.1 cun from the corner of the nail.	Puncture superficially 0.1 inch.
Zhongbai (中白穴, middle-white point)	21	On the back of hand, between the 4th and the 5th metacarpal bone.	Puncture vertically 0.3-0.5 inch.
Zhongchong (中冲 PC9)	21	In the centre of the tip of the middle finger.	Puncture superficially 0.1 inch or prick with a three-edged needle to cause bleeding.

Zhongdu (中渎 GB32)	26	On the lateral aspect of the thigh, 2 cun below Fengshi (GB-31), or 5 cun above the transverse popliteal crease, between m. vastus lateralis and m. biceps femoris.	Puncture vertically 0.7-1.0 inch.
Zhongwan (中脘 REN12)	15	On the anterior midline, 4 cun above the umbilicus.	Puncture perpendicularly 0.5-1.2 inches.
Zhongji (中极 REN3)	15	On the anterior midline, 4 cun below the umbilicus.	Puncture vertically 0.5-1.0 inch. Great care should be taken to puncture the points from Qugu (REN-02) to Shangwan (REN-13) of this meridian in pregnant women.
Zhongzhu (中渚 SJ3)	21	On the dorsum of the hand, in the depression just proximal to the fourth and fifth metacarpophalangeal joints.	Puncture vertically 0.3-0.5 inch.
Zhoubin (筑宾 KID9)	29	5 cun directly above Taixi (KI-3) at the lower end of the belly of m. gastrocnemius, on the line drawn from Taixi (KI-3) to Yingu (KI l0).	Puncture vertically 0.5-0.7 inch.
Zhoujian (肘尖穴, elbow-tip point)	16	on the out tip of elbow	Puncture vertically 0.3-0.5 inch.
Zhouliao (肘髎 LI12)	16	When the elbow is flexed, this point is located in the depression 1 cun proximal to and 1 cun lateral to Quchi L.I.-	Puncture vertically 0.5-1.0 inch.

Zulingqi (足临泣 GB41)	32	In the depression distal to the junction of the 4th and 5th metatarsal bones, on the lateral side of the tendon of m. extensor digitorum longus (branch to little toe).	Puncture vertically 0.3-0.5 inch.
Zusanli (足三里 ST36)	28, 30	Below the knee, 3 cun inferior to Dubi ST-35, one fingerbreadth lateral to the anterior crest of the tibia.	Puncture vertically 0.5-1.2 inches.
Zuqiaoyin (足窍阴 GB44)	32	On the dorsal aspect of the 4th toe, at the junction of lines drawn along the lateral border of the nail and the base of the nail, approximately 0.1 cun from the corner of the nail.	Puncture superficially about 0.1 inch.
Zutonggu (足通谷 UB66)	31, 32	On the lateral side of the foot, in the depression anterior and inferior to the fifth metatarsophalangeal joint.	Puncture vertically 0.2-0.3 inch.

Chapter 4   Acupuncture Points Figures

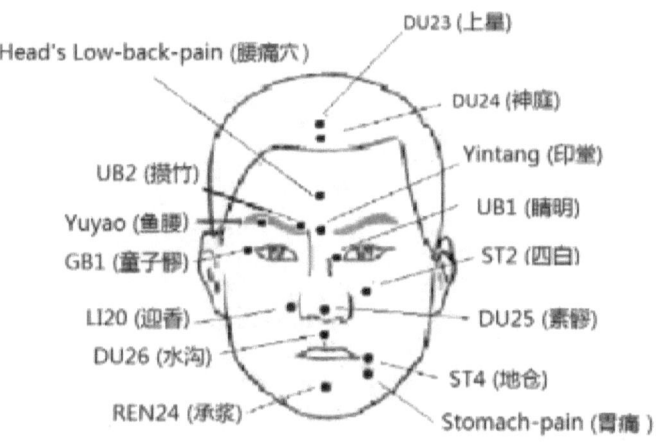

Figure 10. Acupuncture points on face

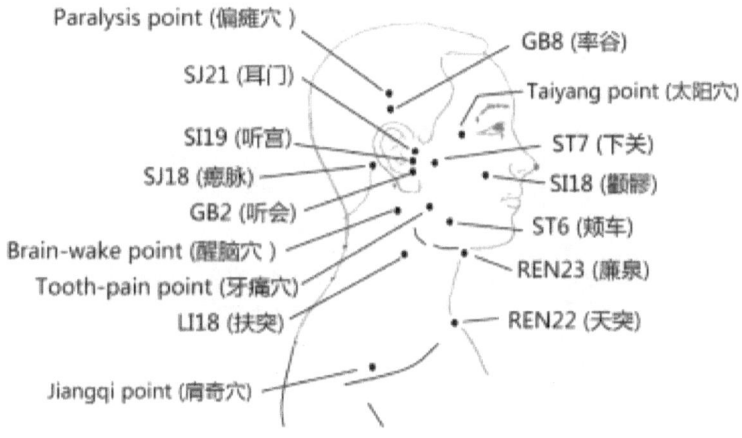

Figure 11. Acupuncture points on side of face

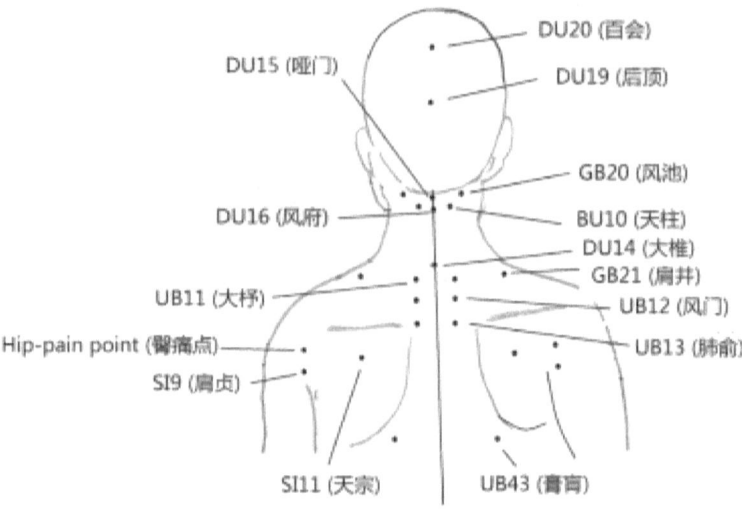

Figure 12. Acupuncture points on back of head and upper back

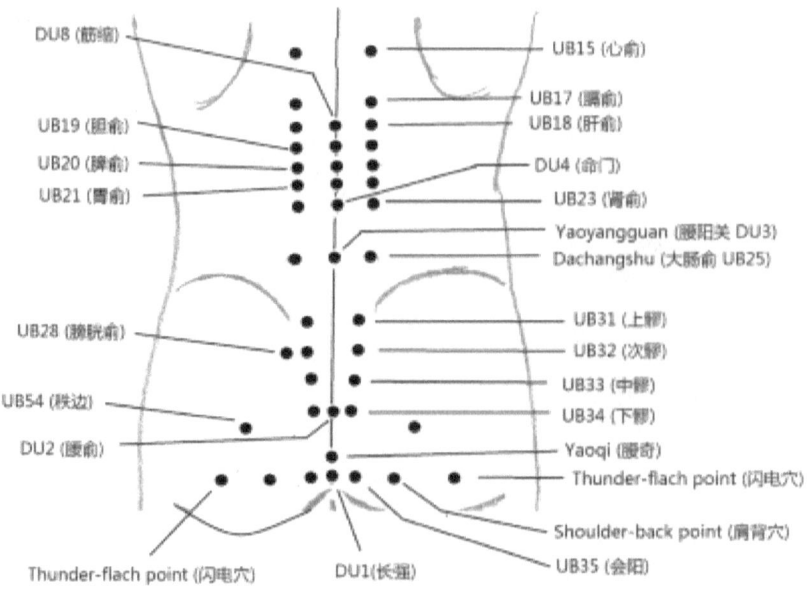

Figure 13. Acupuncture points on back

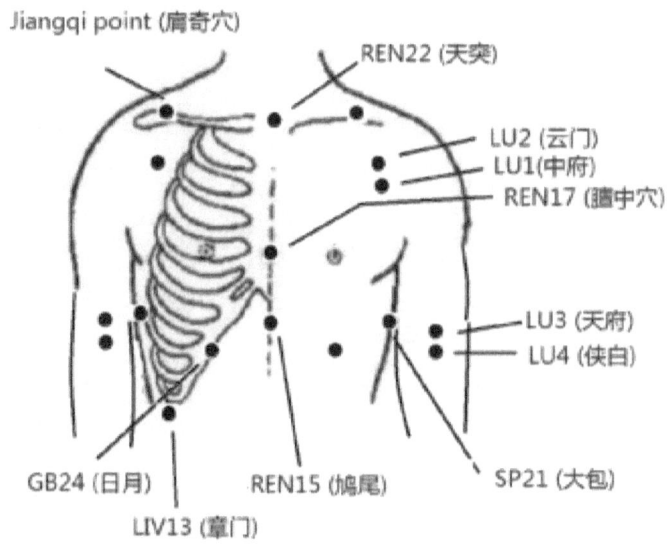

Figure 14. Acupuncture points on upper front body

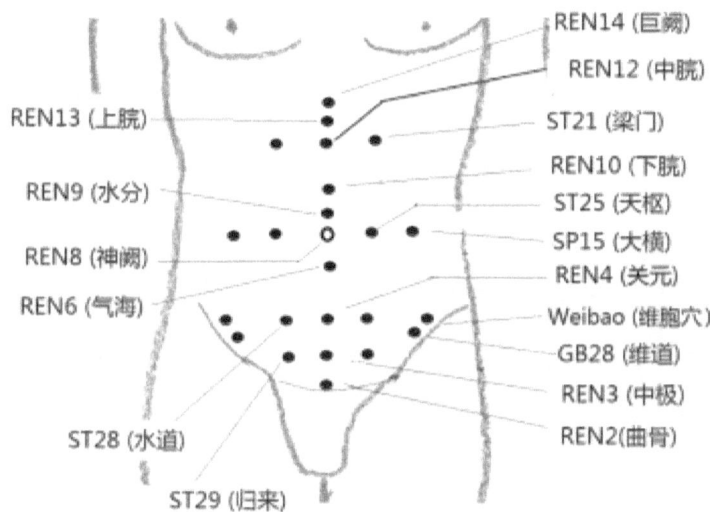

Figure 15. Acupuncture points on lower front of body

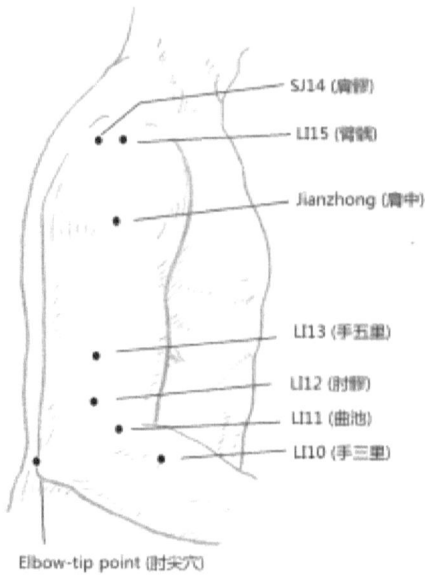

Figure 16. Acupuncture points on upper side of arm

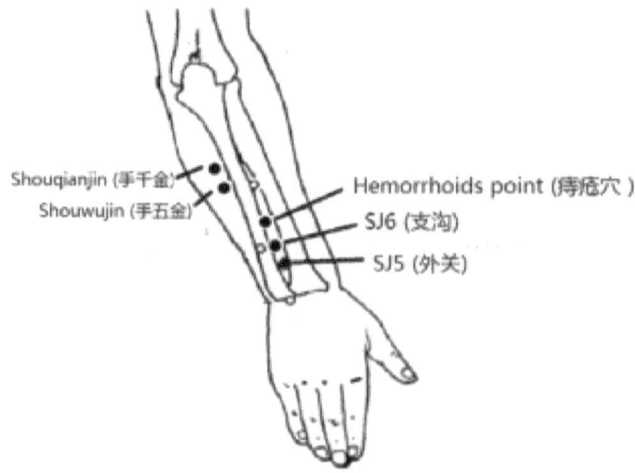

Figure 17. Acupuncture points on back of front arm

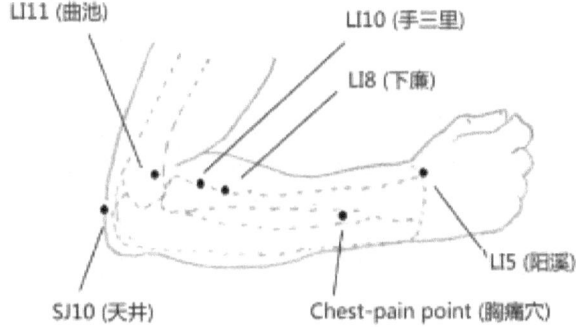

Figure 18. Acupuncture points on back of front arm

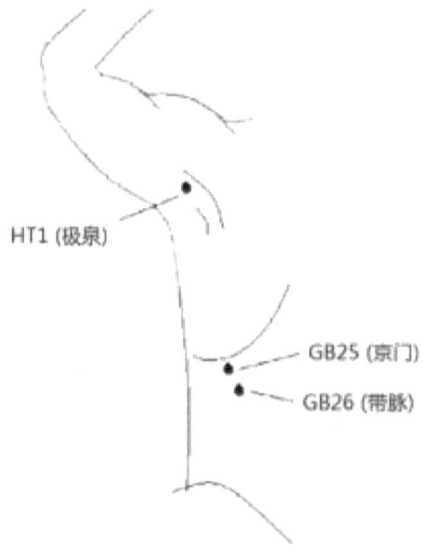

Figure 19. Acupuncture points of HT1, Daomai, and GB25

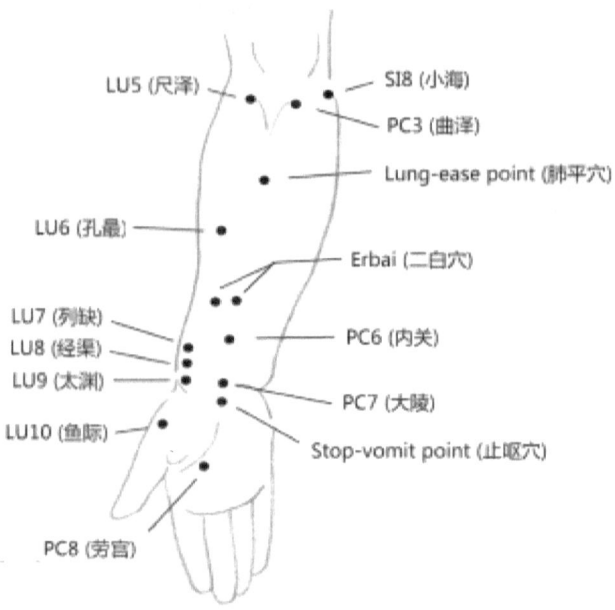

Figure 20. Acupuncture points on inner side of front arm

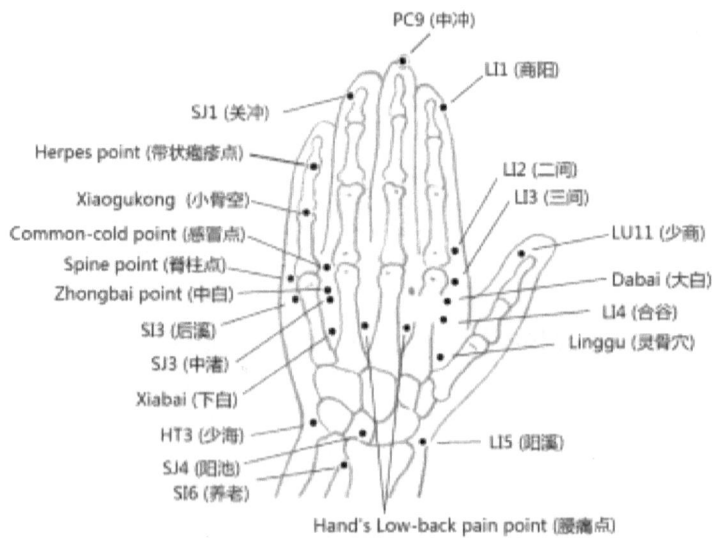

Figure 21. Acupuncture points on back of hand

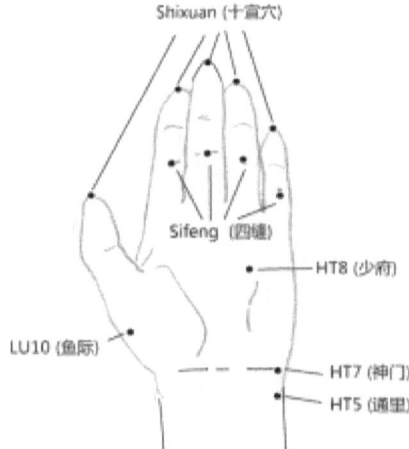

Figure 22. Acupuncture points on palm

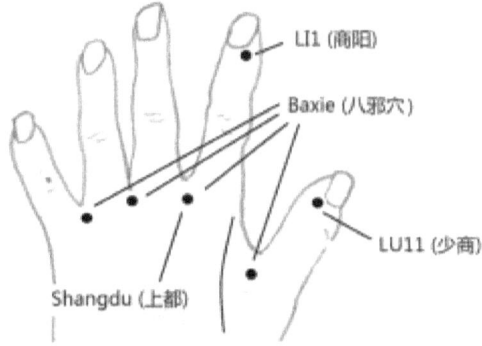

Figure 23. Acupuncture points on back of hand

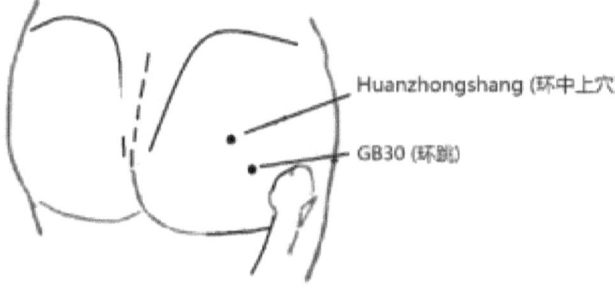

Figure 24. Acupuncture points on hip

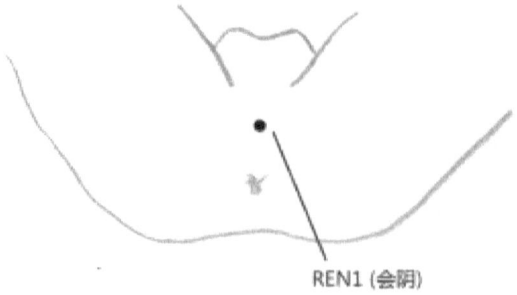

Figure 25. Acupuncture point of REN1

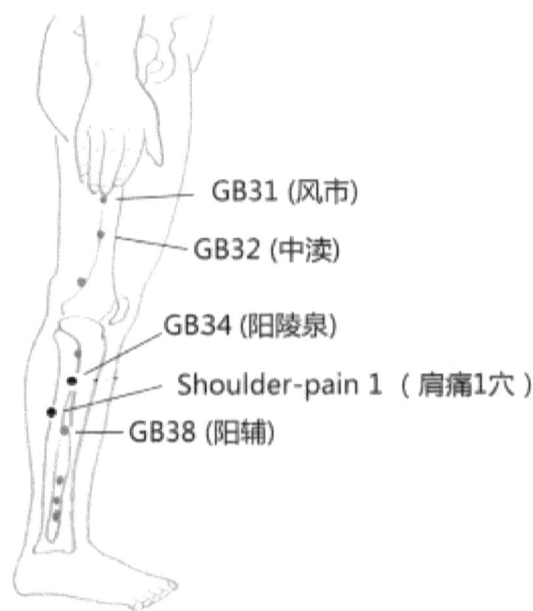

Figure 26. Acupuncture points on side of leg

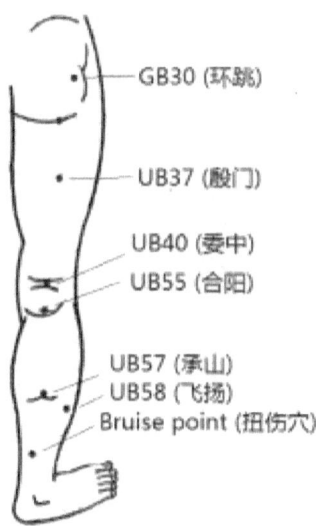

Figure 27. Acupuncture points on back of leg

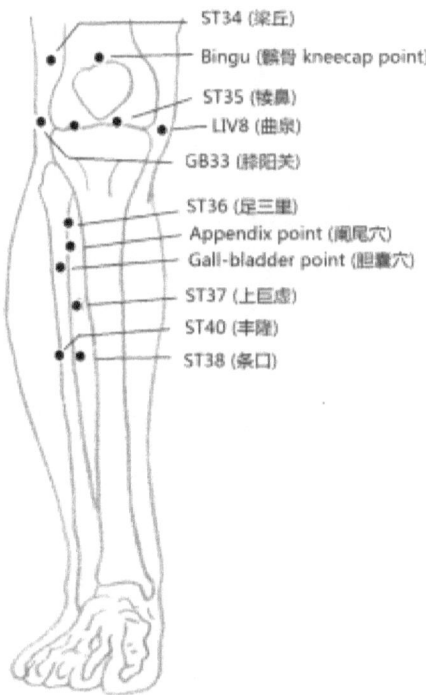

Figure 28. Acupuncture points on front of leg

123

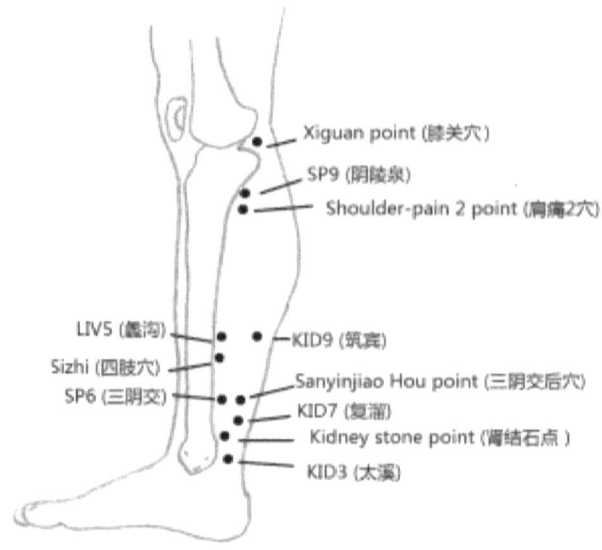

Figure 29. Acupuncture points on inside of leg

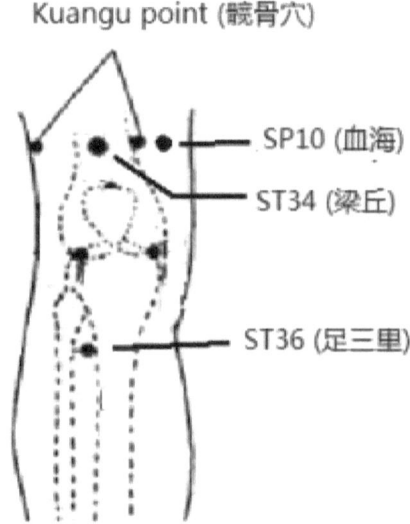

Figure 30. Acupuncture points around the knee

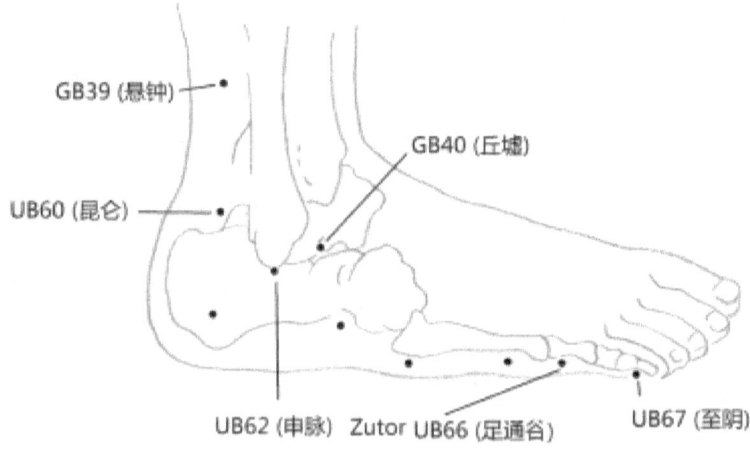

Figure 31. Acupuncture points on side of foot

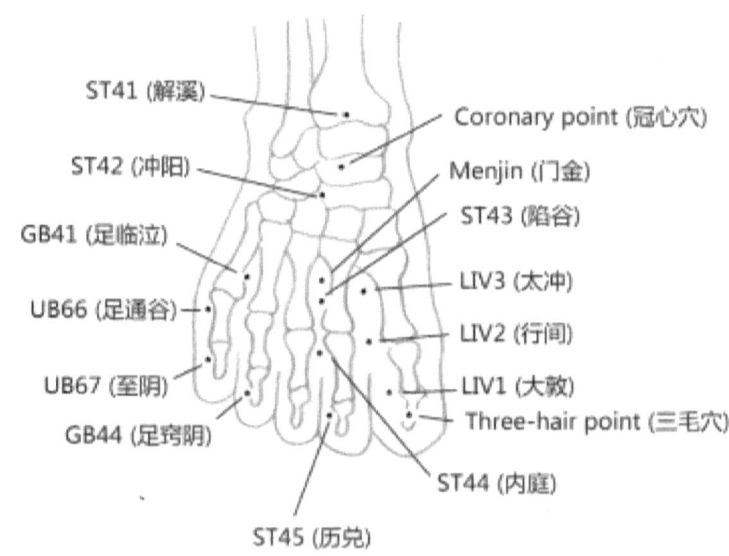

Figure 32. Acupuncture points on back of foot

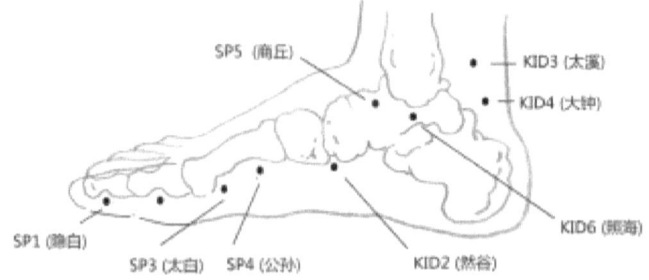

Figure 33. Acupuncture points on inside of foot

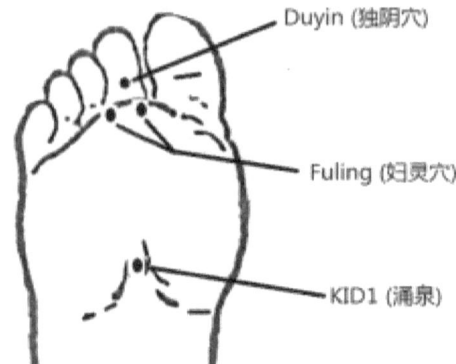

Figure 34. Acupuncture points on sole

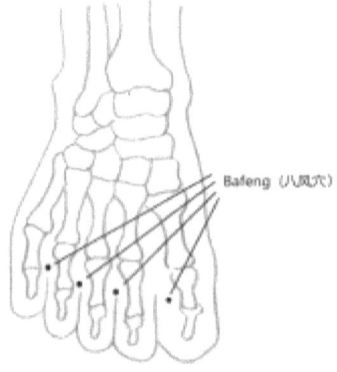

Figure 35. Acupuncture points of Bafeng (eight-wind point)

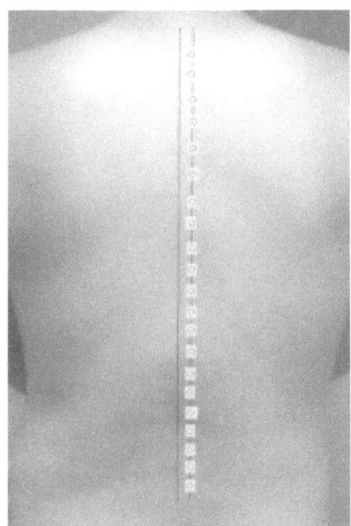

Figure 36. Acupuncture points of Jiaji points (along both sides of the spine)

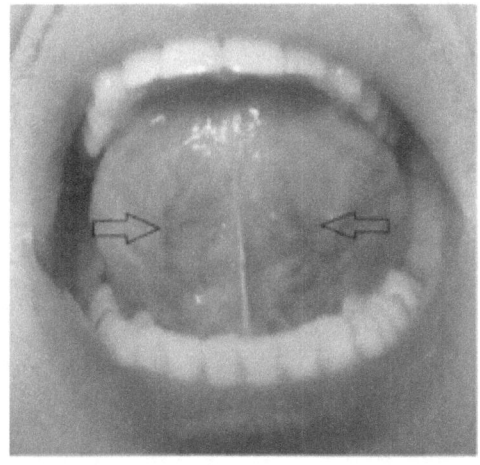

Figure 37. Acupuncture points under the tongue (both sides)

Alphabetic index

Acute and Heavy Dizziness	44
Acute Appendicitis	65
Acute Back Pain	49
Acute Bruise on the Ankle	54
Acute Constipation	74
Acute Diarrhea	74
Acute Gallstones	65
Acute Gastritis	62
Acute Intestinal Obstruction or Enteroparalysis	66
Acute Kidney Stone	66
Acute Knee Pain	53
Acute Mumps	62
Acute Pain in the Mouth, Throat, or Abdomen	59
Acute Pain in the Throat	61
Acute Pain on the Body's Surface	44
Acute Pain on the Elbow	48
Acute Pain on the Heel	55
Acute Sciatic Pain	51
Acute Shoulder Pain	47
Acute Tailbone Pain	52
Acute Urinary Retention	76
Acute Wrist Pain	49
Aphonia	71
Bell's Palsy	45
Bites by Animals or Insects	81
Bites by Bees or Other Insects	81
Bites by Dogs or Other Animals	83
Bites by Snakes	82
Bleeding	21
Bleeding Due to Trauma (beating, car accident, and so on)	21
Bleeding from nose or gums	22
Bleeding from the intestine	23

Bleeding from the lung	22
Bleeding from the stomach	23
Bleeding from the urinary system	24
Bleeding from the Uterus	32
Burns (Fire, Boiling Water, and Similar)	35
Calf Spasm	54
Carbon Monoxide Toxicity	43
Cerebral Concussion	27
Coma	20
Common Cold or Flu	79
Drowning	38
Drunkenness	83
Due to Car Sickness (or Plane Sickness or Boat Sickness)	72
Due to Gastric Disorders	72
Due to Pregnancy	72
Dysmenorrhea	32
Epilepsy	30
Expedite Fetus Delivery	34
Fetus Malposition	33
Fishbone Stuck in Throat	77
Foot Pain	56
Foreign Matter in the Ear	84
Frostbite	36
Gastric Ulcer	64
Gout	56
Gynecology and Obstetrics	32
Headache Due to High Blood Pressure	46
Heart Disease	29
Heart Failure—When the Heart Is About to Stop Beating	30
Heatstroke	42
Heavy Asthma	78
Heavy Cough	68
Hemorrhoids	67
Herpes Zoster	58
Hiccups	70
High Fever	25

Hysteria	31
Incarcerated Hernia	66
Internal Bleeding	22
Migraine	44
Mouth Ulcer	60
Myocardial Infarction and Angina Pectoris4	29
Nausea and Vomiting	72
Neck Stiffness	46
Nocturnal Fretfulness in Infants	34
Panic Attack	30
Retained Placenta	34
Roundworm in Gallbladder	65
Shock	19
Stroke	25
Toothache	59
Trauma	27
Trauma to Abdomen	28
Trauma to Body Muscles	28
Trauma to Chest	27
Trigeminal Neuralgia	45

Our Publications

- More Than Acupuncture
- Acupuncture for Emergencies
- Acupuncture Styles in Current Practice
- What We Can Learn from Acupuncture Research in Western Countries
- Does Nora Five-element Acupuncture Depend mostly on Psychological Effect?

Books are available in Amazon.com

References

51 Yam. "Introduction of the Yin-Yang Nine Acupuncture by Yu Hao." http://www.51yam.com/thread-2 56316-1-1.html.

Bing, Tai. "Experience in the Treatment of Pain and Swelling in Knee." Yanggong Xia de Weixiao. 360 Private Library. http://www.360doc.com/content/12/1016/11/565339_241770042.shtml.

Chinese Medicine. "Acupuncture Treatment of Acute Lumbar Muscle Sprain." Herbalogy. http://www.21nx.com/21nx/html/mifang/waikemifang/gushangke/yaobeisuanto/2012/0926/31905.html.

Chuangxin Yixue. "Marvelous 'Ghost Gate Thirteen-Needle Acupuncture' Therapy." https://read01.com/gRx4kG.html.

Disease Treatment. "Acupuncture Point Treatment of Knee Pain and Foot Pain." http://www.jibingnet.com/waike/jiaotong/14060.asp.

Elderly Healthcare. "Can Acupuncture Treat Feet Pain in Elderly? The Healing Effect of Acupuncture." http://laoren.jiankangzu.com/136215/.

Five-Element Blooming. "New Explanation about Dr. Zhang's Hand-Feet Three-Needle Acupuncture." http://www.360doc.com/content/13/0526/09/11980212_288236524.shtml.

Global Hospitals. "Acupuncture Treatment of Constipation." . http://www.qqyy.com/zhiliao/xhnk/200811/2cf9.html.

He, Guang-Xing, and Yan-Hua Qu. *Mobile Acupuncture Therapy and the Treatment of Pain*. Beijing, China: Xueyuan Press, 2005.

He, Shao-Qi. "Talk about Medicine." Medical Education. http://www.med66.com/html/ziliao/07/67/d2c51ac4b6aa9b39dd1

f6cc4b680289b.html.

He, Xu-Guang and Xing Li. "Clinical Observation on the Effect of Waking-Up-Clear-Mind Acupuncture Therapy in the Treatment of Coma Patients Due to Brain Trauma." *World Health Digest* 47 (2012): 71–72.

Hong, Jie. "Treatment of Tailbone Pain with Acupuncture." http://z.xywy.com/doc/hongjiedr/wenzhang/83-64712.htm.

Hui, Mei-Lan 581. "Treatment of Primary Tailbone Pain with Dong's Mysterious Acupuncture Technique." 360 Private Library. http://www.360doc.com/content/12/0519/17/9844492_212134597.shtml.

Human-Health Lian. "Acupuncture Treatment of Acute Lumbar Muscle Sprain." http://www.360doc.com/content/14/1212/21/15551177_432488983.shtml.

Jiu, Ji-Ling. "Liu Ji Ling New One-Needle Acupuncture." https://v.qq.com/x/page/v0191de3sdh.html.

Laozhongyi. "Treatment of Sciatic with Chinese Medicine." http://www.laozhongyi.net/zhenjiu/zhenjiuzhuanke/waikejihuan/2007-10-22/2425.html.

Liang, Li-Wu, Shen-Tian Song, Ji-Xin Xu, Jun-Qing Lu. *One-Needle Acupuncture*. Beijing, China: Science and Technology Press, 2009.

Lingnan Chinese Herbs. "Which Acupuncture Point Should Be Used in the Treatment of Constipation with Acupuncture?" http://www.tcm360.com/zyly/tszy/159-12965.html.

Lu, Jiang-Ping, En-Qin Zhang, Wei-Xin Jin, Ping Xu. *Acupuncture*. Beijing: Science Press, 1994.

Medical Education. "Good Result in the Treatment of Intestinal Obstruction with Acupuncture." http://www.med66.com/html/ziliao/07/79/ff99dc2d99ab4c337ff158793b47bee6.htm.

Modan. "Emergency Treatment of Drowned Person." Forum of Sunshine Acupuncture, Moxibustion, and Tuina Massage. http://bbs.ygzyxx.com/forum.php?mod=viewthread&tid=7194.

Ni, Hai-Xia. "Chinese Acupuncture." https://www.youtube.com/results?search_query=%E5%80%AA%E6%B5%B7%E5%8E%A6%E9%92%88%E7%81%B8.

One Needle One World. "Jin Three-Needle Acupuncture Therapy." http://baike.baidu.com/view/640926.htm.

Pan, Tong-Xue. "A Review of Acupuncture Treatment of Ankle Bruise." http://blog.sina.com.cn/s/blog_48d11cf1010002i0.html.

Peterjo. "Christ-Western Medicine-Chinese Medicine—Distance Luo Medicine." http://blog.xuite.net/peterjo/diary/69247612-%E5%9F%BA%E7%9D%A3%E4%B8%AD%E8%A5%BF%E9%86%AB%E5%AD%B8-%E9%81%A0%E7%B5%A1%E9%86%AB%E5%AD%B8.

Qyphhh. "Treatment of Acute Lumbar Muscle Sprain with Acupuncture." 360 Private Library. http://www.360doc.com/content/14/0617/17/14765814_387539494.shtml.

Sacred Lotus. "Acupuncture Point and Chart." https://www.sacredlotus.com/go/acupuncture/.

Shen, Yao-Zi. "Treatment of Intestinal Obstruction." In *Yi Bian*, http://yibian.hopto.org/shu/?sid=7788.

Shen, Yao-Zi. "Treatment of Acute Retention of Urine." In *Yi Bian*. http://yibian.hopto.org/shu/?sid=7785.

Shui Na Bai Se. "How Many Lives Can Be Saved? The Emergency Treatment of Drowned People." http://blog.sina.com.cn/s/blog_7a3dc0c9010118fg.html.

Si Yuan. "Si Yuan Balance Method Acupuncture." *Si Yuan Newsletter*. www.siyuanbalance.com/.

Strinkers. "Characteristics of Tang's Balancing Acupuncture System." Forum of Ai Ai Yi. http://bbs.iiyi.com/thread-2548630-1.html.

The Society of Chinese Heath Care. "How to Treat Tailbone Pain with Acupuncture?" Nanjing Acupuncture and Moxibustion School. http://zj.jkpeixun.com/a/zhenjiuzhiliao/20131127/94.html.

The Writing Group for the Rescue of Drowning. *The Rescue of Drowning*. Shanghai, China: Shanghai People's Publishing House, 1972.

Wang, Ben-Zheng. *Bleeding Therapy*. Haerbin, China: Harbin Publishing House, 2003.

Wang, Wen-Yuan. "Wenyuan Balancing Acupuncture Technique." http://www.100md.com/index/0h/d1/0a/16/index.htm.

Wang, Xiao-Yan and Shu-Jun Wu. "Treatment of Persistent Vegetative State after Brain Injury with Waking-Up-Refreshing-Mind Acupuncture Technique." *Chinese J Rehab Med* 21, no. 6 (2006): 547–548.

Wei, Bai-Hai. "Current Clinic Situations in the Treatment of Shock." *Chinese Acupuncture*. 6 (1982): 43–45.

Wu, Shu-Qing. "Introduction of the Experience in Use of 'One-Needle Acupuncture Therapy' Introduced by Han Wen Zhi." 2008 International Conference of Famous Chinese Doctors and Herbalists.

Conference Literature Collection. 2008, Guangzhou, China.

Wu, Xue-Qun. "Electro-Acupuncture Treatment in the Wake-Up of 30 Coma Patients Due to Craniocerebral Trauma." *Chinese Acupuncture & Moxibustion* 25, no. 3 (2005): 200.

Xian Zai Ju Shi. "Special Ways for the Treatment of Knee Pain." http://blog.sina.com.cn/s/blog_6383a68a0102e21g.html.

Xing Lin Ya Shi. "Eight-Word Acupuncture Therapy." 360 Private Library of Xing Lin Ya Shi. www.360doc.com/content/10/0818/09/840524_47041342.shtml.

Xu, Kai-Sheng, Jian-Hua Song, Zhao-Hua Huang, Zhi-Hua Huang, Lu-Chang Yu, Wei-Ping Zheng, Xiao-Shan Chen, Chuang Liu. "Clinical Efficacy Observation of Acupuncture at DU25 (GV25) on Improving Regain of Consciousness from Coma in Severe Craniocerebral Injury." *Chinese Acupuncture & Moxibustion* 34, no. 6 (2014): 529–533.

Xu, Wen-Qi. "Advance in the Treatment of Metatarsalgia with Acupuncture." Doctor's Community. http://www.yishengshequ.com/Info/view/pidl/3/id/5944.html.

Yang Sheng Zhi Dao. "Acupuncture Treatment of Acute Low Back Pain." https://read01.com/QaBEG5.html.

Yang, Shu-Fa and Xi-Chen Wang. "Clinical Rehabilitation Treatment of Patients with Persistent Vegetative State." *Chinese J Rehab Med* 13, no. 2 (1998): 72–74.

Yansheng Zhi Dao. "Which Acupuncture Points Should Be Used for the Treatment of Knee Pain."

Yang, Wei-Jie. *Dong's Qi Acupuncture*. Beijing, China: Ancient Books Publishing House, 1995.

Yang, Yao-Jian. "Influence of Qi and Blood—Tailbone Pain." http://lj.hkej.com/lj2017/healthbeauty/article/id/930844.

Yin Yang House. "Acupuncture Point Location and Chart." Acupuncture.com. https://theory.yinyanghouse.com/acupuncturepoints/x-yuyao.

Yixue Baike. "Acute Urine Retention.". http://www.wiki8.com/jixingniaozhuliu_37439/.

Yu, Qin-Long. "Acupuncture Treatment of Shock in Artificial Abortion Operation." *Jiangsu J TCM* 18, no. 9 (1997): 30.

Zhang, Meng-Chao. "Acupuncture Treatment (String Moxibustion of Zhuang Nationality Medicine) of Herpes Zoster." YouTube. https://www.youtube.com/watch?v=8KGUBo7KrSw.

Zhang, Tian-Sheng, Pei-Rui Nie, Fang Guan and Hong Wen. "Brief Discussion about the 'Yi Tong Zhu Ten' Acupuncture Technique Introduced by Professor Wen Hong." *China Naturopathy*. 22, no. 1 (2014): 8–9.

Zhang, Wei-Wei. "Experienced Recipe for the Treatment of Fishbone Block in Larynx." 360 Private Library. http://www.360doc.com/content/14/0109/14/11726583_343843393.shtml.

Zhang, Xiao-Li and Guang-Ye Song. "Treatment of Coma Patients Due to Severe Brain Trauma with Penetrating-Point Acupuncture." *Chinese Acupuncture* (1994): 303

Zhong Kang Ji Le. "Acupuncture Point Treatment of Sciatic." 360 Private Library. http://www.360doc.com/content/10/0308/11/949724_17972697.shtml.

Zhongyi Shijia. "Foot Back Pain. Bianque Shengying Zhengjiu Yulong Jing." http://www.zysj.com.cn/lilunshuji/bianqueshenyingzhenjiuyulongjing5708/300-2-58.html.

Zhou, Zhi-Jie, Ke-Jing Yin, Cai-Ping Han, Fu-Hui Zhang, Xiong-Cang Wu, Xiao-Jian Jiang. *Acupuncture Treatment of Clinic Emergency*. Xian, China: Shaanxi Science and Technology Press, 1988.
https://books.google.ca/books?id=h4LF1DAFYTkC&pg=PA117&lpg=PA117&dq=%E6%BA%BA%E6%B0%B4%E9%92%88%E7%81%B8&source=bl&ots=9giRzrp-Ol&sig=u-IsdrInpigADdJFWlyFPWFNEVQ&hl=en&sa=X&ved=0ahUKEwjXu8amuPjXAhUE3WMKHRAoBtUQ6AEIWDAL#v=onepage&q=%E6%BA%BA%E6%B0%B4%E9%92%88%E7%81%B8&f=false.

(All online references are cited before August 2, 2017.)

www.ingramcontent.com/pod-product-compliance
Lightning Source LLC
Chambersburg PA
CBHW031422210526
45464CB00005B/2012